The Changing Context of Social-Health Care: Its Implications for Providers and Consumers

The Changing Context of Social-Health Care: Its Implications for Providers and Consumers

Helen Rehr, DSW
Gary Rosenberg, PhD
Editors

The Haworth Press
New York • London

The Haworth Press, Inc., 10 Alice Street, Binghamton, NY 13904-1580
EUROSPAN/Haworth, 3 Henrietta Street, London WC2E 8LU England

Library of Congress Cataloging-in-Publication Data

The Changing context of social-health care : its implications for providers and consumers / edited by Helen Rehr and Gary Rosenberg.
    p.   cm.
    Papers from the Fifth Doris Siegel Memorial Colloquium, held Oct. 20-21, 1988, at the Mount Sinai Medical Center and hosted by the Doris Siegel Memorial Fund Committee.
    Includes bibliographical references and index.
    ISBN 1-56024-143-8 (acid free paper). — ISBN 1-56024-144-6 (pbk.)
    1. Social medicine — United States — Congresses. 2. Medical policy — United States — Congresses. I. Rehr, Helen. II. Rosenberg, Gary. III. Siegel, Doris, d. 1971. IV. Doris Siegel Memorial Fund Committee. V. Doris Siegel Memorial Colloquium (5th : 1988 : Mount Sinai Medical Center)
RA418.3.U6C43   1991
362.1′0973 — dc20
                                         91-2250
                                            CIP

The Changing Context
of Social-Health Care:
Its Implications
for Providers
and Consumers

CONTENTS

PART IV: CONCLUSIONS AND RECOMMENDATIONS

APPENDIXES

INDEX

The Changing Context of Social-Health Care: Its Implications for Providers and Consumers

ABOUT THE EDITORS

Helen Rehr, DSW, is Professor of Community Medicine (Social Work) Emerita at The Mount Sinai School of Medicine, CUNY. She is the author of over eighty publications dealing with a range of social-health issues, professional accountability, and quality assurance. She has been honored with many awards, including election to the Hunter College Hall Fame, The Ida M. Cannon Award and most recently with the First Knee/Wittman Lifetime Achievement Award of the National Association of Social Work. She also serves on a number of editorial boards.

Gary Rosenberg, PhD, is the Edith J. Baerwald Professor of Community Medicine (Social Work) and Senior Vice President at The Mount Sinai Medical Center, New York City. He is past President of the Society for Hospital Social Work Directors of the American Hospital Association. Dr. Rosenberg has been elected to the Hunter College Hall of Fame and has received the Distinguished Alumni Award from Adelphi University and the Founders Day Award from New York University. In addition, he is a Fellow in the Brookdale Center on Aging and a recipient of the Ida M. Cannon Award of the Society for Hospital Social Work Directors.

Preface

On behalf of The Doris Siegel Memorial Committee, it is with great pride that I welcome you to the Fifth Doris Siegel Memorial Colloquium. The Mount Sinai Medical Center is honored to host these colloquia, which, since 1973, have contributed — through critical presentations by leaders in health care, workshop deliberations, and their publications — to knowledge regarding the most timely social-health care issues in the country.

Doris' friends and colleagues established the Fund to memorialize her outstanding commitment to social work services and her love for quality medical care. The mission of The Doris Siegel Fund is "to encourage and support social work in its efforts to enhance the social effectiveness of health and medical care."

I am especially honored to host these proceedings today. I met Doris in the late 1960s and have known of her inspirational leadership through her writings, presentations at conferences and, in particular, in being able to count her contributions to Mount Sinai in innovative social work programs and in enhanced health care services. Doris was committed to equity and justice for all people in their access to social-health services.

Today's program will deal with the challenges we face as we confront the changes in medicine and in health care delivery and try to understand their implications for what must be done in this country to secure access for all of us to quality social-health services. Today, in pursuing the topic "The Changing Context of Social-Health Care: Its Implications for Providers and Consumers," we have the help of presentations by two outstanding thinkers in the

field and the deliberations of leading social and health care professionals.

We shall again be proud to publish these proceedings.

Gary Rosenberg, PhD
Executive Secretary
The Doris Siegel Memorial Fund Committee
and
Edith J. Baerwald Professsor
of Community Medicine (Social Work)
Mount Sinai School of Medicine
City University of New York

Greetings

It is a pleasure to welcome you to Mount Sinai and to the Doris Siegel Memorial Colloquium. Doris Siegel was an exceptional and outstanding person at Mount Sinai. She was beloved and respected both here and nationally for her leadership, her compassion, and her professional wisdom. Doris Siegel served as the first Edith J. Baerwald Professor of Community Medicine at Mount Sinai. As such she held what was, and still is, the only chair of social work in an American medical school. In that role, Ms. Siegel—with her social work faculty in the medical school's Division of Social Work of the Department of Community Medicine—brought a psycho-social-environmental orientation to service, research, and education. Her work was encouraged and supported by the able and strong leadership of Dr. Kurt W. Deuschle, the department's chairman.

This is the fifth Colloquium dedicated to Doris Siegel. Her ideals played an exceptionally important role in both the academic and the clinical, as well as in the managerial aspects of the institution.

In the early 1960s the hospital honored the contributions of social work and nursing by electing their leaders—both women—to serve on the Medical Board of Mount Sinai where each reinforced the Judeo-Christian tenet of humanitarianism and social responsibility to those who "have not." Social work and nursing continue to make invaluable contributions at the highest administrative and program levels.

I am told Ms. Siegel was a Bostonian and carried with her to Pittsburgh, Washington D.C., and Mount Sinai that "je sais faire" that is characteristic of all Bostonian leaders. Eleanor Clarke of Massachusetts General, a colleague and friend of Doris, was also outstanding, and I suspect my own drive comes out of that region as well.

It is clear to me that persons who achieve a key role in an academic center become valued commodities. They bring, as Doris

xiii

Siegel did, a social system's perspective to their management approach. In present day academic health centers a social organizational approach is a must. These leaders bring a focus on people rather than just on dollars and that is a welcome change. Dollars are important — it is important for me to say that, someone on the Board of Trustees is no doubt here. They bring, beyond the focus on people as individuals, a focus on the community. My own view is that academic health centers will increasingly need to relate to the community that surrounds them. We have been wonderfully lucky to have had the leadership of Doris Siegel followed by her successor, Dr. Helen Rehr, and now Dr. Gary Rosenberg — all of whom have brought commitment and outstanding contributions to the Mount Sinai Medical Center.

Dr. John W. Rowe, President
Mount Sinai School of Medicine and
The Mount Sinai Medical Center

Tribute

As you have heard, this is the Fifth Colloquium in tribute to Doris Siegel. There are those among you who remember her well and those who wonder who she was. It is my privilege to tell you a little about this remarkable woman, who was an outstanding professional and a very special human being.

She was responsible for developing one of the country's best social work departments, and as you have heard, was the first Edith J. Baerwald Professor, occupying the only endowed chair in social work in an American school of medicine.

Before coming to Mount Sinai she had directed the social work department at Montefiore Hospital in Pittsburgh. She then became a consultant for the United States Children's Bureau and was responsible for major contributions in planned services throughout the country for physically and developmentally disabled children and their families.

The social-health programs she initiated at Mount Sinai reflect her advocacy for the needy, her ability to work for change, and her entrenched belief in the importance of collaboration among health care professionals.

Doris was a native of Boston. She always felt that that gave her something special—something more than the rest of us had. She certainly had a sense of self, conviction in her beliefs, and an abiding determination to defend her social commitments. These attributes, coupled with her warmth for people, enabled her to instill in others love for a cause and for service.

She was a sort of earth mother, who was always there for her staff and for her colleagues. She worked harder than anyone else and we wanted to work hard to reach the goals she set.

Doris was both challenging and supportive. I remember shortly after I arrived at Mount Sinai she asked me to assess the department's program and status—that was 1955. I did and one of my recommendations was to exchange untrained workers for trained ones. After hearing me out, she said "Dolly"—many of you will remember she addressed you that way—"that's a brilliant analysis, but why don't we try to bring people to the level we want. Those who will want to join us will do something, and those who don't will probably leave." How right she was! Most staff rose to expectations with special educational programs and schooling opportunities for which she secured assistance from the Mount Sinai Auxiliary Board. The others left over time. Her commitment was to "high staff morale," which she felt was critical for a quality program, a major administrative principle that holds today.

Doris was the most courageous woman I have known. She was also creative. These characteristics made her an initiator and supporter of new programs, such as the pioneering Patient Representative Service, Social-Health Advocates, and a range of community networking programs to enhance social-health services for our patients and agency clients. These activities, created in the 1960s, made her a thinker and a doer ahead of her times. At her investiture to the Edith J. Baerwald Chair in 1969, she said social work and medicine have responsibility for "reaching out more aggressively not only to those we serve, but to those whom we should serve." Thus she keynoted the access problem with which we wrestle today. Her abiding sense of the importance of collaboration between professional and lay groups was a moving force in making her beloved Auxiliary Board the vital member of the Mount Sinai community it is today. She was also a prime factor in the development of the hospital's Community Board.

Doris was a generous, giving person. She constantly wove little squares—we called them "latkes"—which ultimately became beautiful afghans for her friends. We would tease her about cooking huge batches of food so she could invite people for "leftovers." She had friends all over the country and was admired, trusted, and loved by them. It is they who have made The Doris Siegel Memorial Fund a reality, making possible these colloquia on key social-health issues. Doris would have loved these meetings. She was committed to the highest quality in social-health care and to reaching the best in people.

These colloquia are Mount Sinai's and social work's tribute to this very outstanding woman. To date they have addressed:

1. the contributions from interprofessional collaboration;
2. ethical dilemmas in social work and medicine;
3. milestones in social work and medicine that have and can contribute to change; and
4. problems and solutions in access to care.

All the colloquia proceedings have been published and can be found in professional schools throughout the country.

Today's forum "The Changing Context of Social-Health Care: Its Implications for Providers and Consumers" follows in this tradition. It is a subject that would appeal to Doris' expectations for contributing to knowledge to enhance human services.

Helen Rehr, DSW
Professor of Community Medicine Emerita
Mount Sinai School of Medicine
City University of New York

Part I

Introduction

Introduction

Helen Rehr

The Doris Siegel Memorial Fund Committee (see Appendix A) convened in 1987 to recommend a fifth colloquium that would deal with a key social-health issue that affects the availability and the quality of health care in the country. A sub-committee was created (see Appendix B) to plan and implement a program to take place in 1988 in keeping with the mission of the Fund, which ties social work and medicine together in their efforts to enhance the social effectiveness of health and medical care.

In 1987 a number of changes occurred in the constituency of the committee. Most significant was the appointment of Dr. Gary Rosenberg as Executive Secretary to succeed Dr. Helen Rehr, who had retired after years of committed service in the development of colloquia, which had received professional recognition for their contribution to knowledge in the social-health care field. Dr. Rehr joined Dr. Rosenberg and Mrs. Bess Dana, a member of the committee from its inception and a former student and friend of Doris', in spearheading the fifth colloquium with the assistance of the sub-committee for planning.

At an early meeting in 1987 a series of topics, which were of great concern to professionals in health care, were raised. These were:

— Chronic Illness: the range of chronic illnesses, the populations at risk, affordability and access to care for all Americans, availability of care, and new services and their quality. A critical issue to which the three planners gave serious thought was the need to view the social costs and consequences of chronic

---

Helen Rehr, DSW, is Professor of Community Medicine Emerita, Mount Sinai School of Medicine, City University of New York.

illness to individuals and their families, with particular emphasis on the roles of social work, medicine and nursing;
— Interprofessionalism Revisited: the first Doris Siegel Colloquium had offered an inspirational program on the values of, but also the central difficulties in achieving true interprofessionalism given the system of health care in its specialized and departmentalized formats. There were many in those earlier deliberations who opted for cooperative interrelationships as needed, rather than on-going collaboration and team relationships as the more realistic and valued way to serve patients;
— Deregulation of Health Care: the impact of the fee-for-service marketplace, competition among health care facilities, and the new reimbursement programs by governmental bodies to hospitals; the costs of deregulation and its effects on care in economic, social service, and quality terms, as well as in institutional responses to key social-health issues, access, in particular;
— Health Care Professionals: the new and traditional practitioners and their changing relationships to medical institutions; new technologies, new demands, new actors in health care such as ethicists, risk managers, economists, and old actors in new roles such as nurse clinicians and clinical pharmacists; the effects of changing health care in institutions on health care professionals.

When the sub-committee met in the late spring of 1987 to develop a theme for the colloquium, the discussion ranged along the topics outlined above as well as others. The sub-committee deliberated on what it saw as the most critical issues for health planning over the next five years. The members understood that while these issues were particular to the New York City area, they were relevant for all in a national context, and planning to deal with them was imperative. The following were noted without setting any priorities:

— Reduce the impact of the financial and political crises on the health care system;
— Regional needs assessments are essential, to be followed quickly by appropriate resource allocations;

— Assure access to health care for the disenfranchised, underinsured, uninsured, and marginal groups;
— Deal with the AIDS crisis in service and in short and long term prevention;
— Tackle long term care needs in appropriate "at home" and institutional services;
— Deal with the homeless at multiple levels;
— Face the high technology factor in cost-effectiveness terms;
— Deal with infant mortality in the inner cities, and make available and reachable pre-natal and infant care;
— Deal with substance abuse problems at both the service and prevention levels;
— Make mental health services more readily available and realistically set to needs.

The discussion on these subjects noted the need for technical analysis through studies to give the public and the policy makers information for policy and program deliberations. Serious concern was registered about the many cutbacks in federally funded programs and the imposed major shift to state and local support. On the other hand, the members believed that health care planning should be regionally based, but with adequate financial underpinning at all government levels. There was recognition that both public and private resources would be essential in any resolution. The concern in regard to health care professionals was that they are usually in reactive positions. They need to become pro-active, to assume advocacy positions after becoming adequately informed. The sub-committee openly recognized that coalitions of professional and consumer groups, along with other forces, such as industry, insurance, and government representation would be essential to achieve broad-based community involvement. The group recognized there could be danger as single issue organizations or groups would participate, but they also supported the right of all issues to be heard in order to develop strategic priorities. It was noted that a major requirement, in addition to studies of selected situations, would be educational changes at many levels. Education at the public level would require political and professional investment, while educational changes in the curricula of the health care professions would be a major undertaking.

How could these major concerns be addressed in a one day forum? The sub-committee struggled to set subject priorities which would be meaningful for today and tomorrow and would serve the health care providers, community, and the public.

Issues for Discussion: Suggested Guidelines

In addressing the impact of the changing health care environment on health care professionals and the consumers of their services, the sub-committee members thought the speakers' content and workshop deliberations (which were being recommended again for this colloquium) could identify the many changes in health care while attempting to deal with the consequences of the reallocation of resources. The subject was both present and future oriented and would allow for an analysis of the current state of institutional care, the changes foreseen and the impact on both providers and consumers. The sub-committee recommended that opportunity should be provided for projections for education of the professions, for services needed and for resource allocation. Factors which have affected institutional change would need to be addressed. New organizations and systems of health care would be identified, as well as the commercialization of care via for-profit hospitals versus the non-profit municipal, voluntary, and teaching institutions. The solo practice of medicine versus group practice, including HMO's and PPO's, could be discussed in the context of how these, as well as new systems of care, affected the health care professional. The "who" and the "how" of preparation for these changes of practitioners, and, as important, of consumers, would be major concerns.

As we looked at the subject and attempted to title it, as well as to identify what we wanted our speakers to address, a series of questions surfaced:

— Do we want to learn the adaptations and the shapings of health care today and tomorrow?
— Are there conflicting expectations between providers and consumers? Can there be a true partnership in health care?
— Should geriatric care and rehabilitation in particular, be primary social work services or at the least, a social-health service? How should functions be differentiated by the various health care professionals?

— If hospitals continue to be accredited by the State and the Joint Commission on Accreditation, who should accredit or hold accountable the different health care professionals?

— DRG's, CON's, and other financial constraints have affected the medical institutions in reimbursement and in innovations; how have they affected regional public health care needs?

— What needs to be done to deal with the public's continuing distrust of the medical profession and the institutions?

— What responsibilities do the health care professions have to project needed reform of delivery? The professions tend to follow the health care delivery system; should they lead based on their understanding of need?

As we focused on the significance of the questions, we believed we should seek speakers who could relate to the impact of changes on the consumer and the provider, and their relationship to each other. We would ask our speakers to give position papers which would address the following:

— "What do you think are the most critical social-health issues today?"

— "What are your expectations of the health care professions, and other providers in dealing with these issues?"

— "What are the effects of government policies (or no policies) on providers and on consumers?"

— "What should be our social-health policies and offerings in services, in research, and in education for the health care professions?"

Finally, there was consensus and the recommended topic was: "The Changing Context of Social-Health Care: Its Implications for Providers and Consumers."

The sub-committee endorsed a plan that called for two speakers in an afternoon forum, open to the public, and a series of workshops to deal with selected aspects of the subject. The workshop was seen as a place to raise the critical issues in greater depth, adding to what might be forthcoming in the presentations. No one believed that workshop discussions would bring out finite solutions, but members thought they would provide for interaction on ideas for the future. They recognized the 21st century is almost upon us. Their concern was that our country is without a sound national health policy. American political action tends to support incremental changes, but not within a comprehensive design as exists in several westernized countries.

They speculated the next ten years were unlikely to bring much in the way of new programs either by federal or state governments unless these activities would be self-supporting. Their expressed hopes were for holding the line on health care expenditures as against the fear of further cutbacks. In any case they were morally committed to a public policy of access to health care for all Americans.

The sub-committee arrived quickly at its choice of speakers. It was clear to all that the individual most knowledgeable to address the changing health care environment and its impact on providers was Dr. Dennis O'Leary, President of the Joint Commission for Accreditation of Health Organizations. The speaker who was first choice to advocate for consumers was the outspoken critic of the health care systems in this country, Emily Friedman, Contributing Editor, *Hospitals*, *Medical World News*, *Health Care Forum Journal,* and *Health Business*. Both accepted.

We next considered the format for the workshops. The workshops would follow the forum, taking place the next day from 9 a.m. to 1 p.m. It was our suggestion that there be five workshops composed of a mix of 10 or more health care professionals from medicine, nursing, social work, health care economics, and sociology. There should be two co-leaders: a doctor and social worker, and a recorder for each. In order to assure discussion in-depth among workshop participants, the sub-committee decided to request "think" pieces from a selected number of invited guests. These would be a three or four page written statement on a given topic resulting in a 10 minute presentation by the author. An invitational presentation, albeit brief, could assure that those from a distance could represent their institutions at the colloquium.

The Forum and Workshops

The Colloquium was held on the afternoon of October 20, and the morning of October 21, 1988 at The Mount Sinai Medical Center. The plenary session was attended by more than 200 people drawn from the range of professions in the health care field, and from the lay and consumer public known to the institution.

Dr. Gary Rosenberg, Executive Secretary of the Committee, opened the Fifth Doris Siegel Memorial Colloquium. He introduced Dr. John W. Rowe, the newly appointed President of the Medical Center, who welcomed the audience and paid tribute to Doris Siegel as an advocate for quality health care. He noted their similarity of interests — the linking of a social systems perspective to the management of clinical care. He also commented on his commitment to the belief that academic health centers, such as Mount Sinai, have a need to relate to the neighboring community and to serve it well. This was a Doris Siegel tenet. Dr. Rosenberg then introduced Dr. Helen Rehr, recognizing her past contributions as the Fund's Executive Secretary to the Doris Siegel Colloquia, and as his friend and mentor. Dr. Rehr, a friend and colleague of Doris for 20 years, extolled her as a friend, but also for her major contributions to social work at Mount Sinai and to the field. Dr. Rosenberg introduced Dr. Dennis O'Leary as the first speaker and Emily Friedman as second.

Dr. O'Leary's topic was "Health Care Today and Tomorrow." He noted that in spite of all the turbulence in our society and in our health care system, people call for the highest quality health care to be made available to those in need of services. He reminded us that even though the United States represents an affluent society, fiscal constraints have become necessary and resources have become finite. We are a consumption oriented society, uniquely preoccupied with the "soma" that has led to a major emphasis on specialty medicine while concerned with the quality of life. Government supported programs of the past have led to an expanded health care system, incremental entitlements, and a burst of technology. The government had to face that it could not afford to pay for all that had been promoted. It moved to instituting deregulation, shifting payment to others (patients and providers), encouraging competition in the medical arena, and promulgating packages of services as preferable, with incentives given to provide less care than more. Competition was driven by price; quality of care became a serious issue as a result of sharp cost containment measures. As malpractice suits grew in number, professional accountability became a number one public and political issue as professional peer self-assessment seemed not to work.

In spite of the problems we face, Dr. O'Leary was optimistic about the future. He saw the patient as the "center" in care, and he believed that planning health care services will continue to have high priority in our society. The care will be more diversified and more specialized calling for more specialists. However, he believed it will be team based and will have quality assurance assessment expectations. All institutional and provider care will be required to have a quality assurance plan for performance geared to satisfaction by both the client and provider. While care will not be perceived in terms of perfection, it will be seen in an atmosphere calling for continuous improvement in performance and in programs.

The challenge for tomorrow, Dr. O'Leary said, is a need for people to work together and to do better tomorrow what we are doing today. If management of patient care is to be effective, it needs good information and data — clinical indicators based on performance. Information serves as the vehicle for raising questions about quality, and for pointing practitioners and planners in a direction essential to improve quality of care. He believed that ultimately as the consumer of care passes judgment based on understanding quality, the future will have to be fluid and open to change and new opportunities.

Emily Friedman followed with a talk entitled "Patients as Partners: The Changing Health Care Environment." Peppered with delicious yet appropriately placed witticisms, Friedman delivered a volatile speech touching on those issues of central concern to the American public and to the consumer/patient as the direct recipient of health care services. She reminded us that it is not true that everyone who gets into the health care system gets equal or the same care. She followed with data highlighting the "access" issue we must all face. The number of Americans who are underinsured, uninsured, and uncovered by Medicaid cutbacks is growing daily. Hospitals, which doled out uncompensated care in the past, are no longer able to continue because of the payment system imposed on them. Those people who are uncovered do not have access and delay care. When they reach emergency rooms, care can be too late and extraordinarily expensive, more so than any service therapeutically or preventively administered in early access. When Americans are polled they overwhelmingly support some form of universal insurance. Ms. Friedman went on to raise the current personnel shortage problem all institutions are facing—especially nurses. Moreover, she claimed not only is there a shortage, but there is a gender change. Women who have been the backbone of medical institutions in menial and in powerless roles are now claiming more influential positions as well as seeking different attitudes and behaviors from male physicians who have dominated the health care field. Women are entering the field of medicine and health care management, and, along with Blacks and Hispanics will make a claim for leadership. As the question of how to "pay" doctors will be raised over and over again, physicians will take to showing their differences among the various specialties, as each claims greater importance and a greater rate of reimbursement. Ms. Friedman believed the "pecking" order will change among specialties, and a new power base for nurses will arise. Health care professionals and quasi-professionals will redefine their working roles.

Ms. Friedman moved to quality of care as the third critical issue and evoked a range of perceptions of that factor depending on who defines it. She described a major change from one's own assessment of quality to that of drawing on a range of information and data collected, and made public. She described what is happening in health care—the abuse and the misuse by providers and their institutions. Consumers and payers have begun a questioning of procedures, practices, and services that will lead all of us to expect quality of care and sound outcomes in the future.

Rationing is another concern Ms. Friedman raised. "Who will decide who gets what?" is the complicated question that we will have to answer. But who will make the determination—the providers or the consumers? While she recognized that the consumers have begun to make a key place for themselves in both the care and planning arenas, providers are still in charge of information, a fact that will tend to give them greater dominance. Ms. Friedman worried most about the payers since dollar availability tends to control coverage. She projected that resolutions of this issue, and others, really should fall to a true partnership between providers with their patients, and the consumer public. However, a true partnership will require a major shift in the public's current view of medicine (and health care) and medicine's self image, before finally, a meaningful trust of each other can occur.

As noted, each workshop was to be set in motion by a "think" piece on selected subjects presented by leaders in the health care field to other leaders. Given the subject of a changing environment and the impact on providers and consumers, the sub-committee arrived at workshop topics as follows:

1. Promoting the scope and reach of clinical social-health services;
2. Organization and management of social-health resources, including their financing;
3. Program and policy planning; the effects of deregulation versus regulation;
4. Education of the health care professions and the functions of inter- and multi-professional relationships;
5. Systematic research and evaluations, and strategies to achieve these.

There were a number of sub-themes we believed were generic to all or most of the workshops. These were noted as follows:

— collaborative relationships among health care professionals;
— engagement of the consumer;
— reconciling the past, present and future;
— equating cost-effectiveness with optimum social-health outcomes;
— impact of the auspices of health care programs, and of the range of reimbursement and financing patterns;
— impact of the changing nature of health care problems and of the changing characteristics of populations at risk.

The "think" pieces, which covered the sub-themes relevant to the five workshops, were presented by their authors under the direction of the leaders, and a recorder (see Appendix C). Leaders and recorders joined together in providing a written report on the content and proceedings of the given workshop discussion, and then joined with others in a reprise and assessment of each of the workshop deliberations. Bess Dana's synthesis of those discussions appears in these proceedings (see Part 3) revealing the in-depth discussion of all participants (see Appendix D), their ability to come to some conclusions, and to identify the areas that warrant more study and more deliberations.

A brief summary of the key comments and findings which derived from each of the five workshops follows:

I. The Clinical/Personal Health Care Systems group registered the concern that the patient/consumer is still missing as a care "partner." The members deliberated regarding how to bring the consumer into the equation. They worried that technology was taking precedence over humanitarianism. Team care was seen as critical and effective, but strain among team members was identified as still prevalent, in particular nurses to doctors. The belief that a social-health model of care was needed in the future was noted. Prevention is a must, but not an "end-all." Sick care services will always be required. A shift from the predominance of the doctor, to a leadership role for the different social-health care professional appropriate to the needs of the patient was forecast. They also urged that more credence than currently exists be given to applied research relevant to clinical needs and practitioners' performance.

II. The Organization and Management group touched on the micro-services available to given populations, the effect of collaborative relationships among health care professionals on the care of the individual, plus the impact of auspice on services and thus on consumers. When collaboration is not available, there is a negative impact on the quality and comprehensiveness of care an individual receives. Professionals need positive and respectful attitudes toward each other in order to achieve positive patient service. On the other hand, as health care professionals deal with the most severe of socially negative diseases, their own powerlessness surfaces, leaving them unresponsive to work with these difficult situations and with each other toward planned and preventive services. Dollars play the most critical part in today's service delivery. Availability and access are affected with the trend to shift costs from government and industry on to the consumer.

III. The Policy, Planning and Regulation group affirmed very early the need for universal health care coverage. Their discussion concentrated on resource allocation while drawing on current ethical and service dilemmas. They identified the current conflict in the provision of services for the elderly at the price of children's care. They asked how society will deal with the huge number of the Americans suffering from chronic disease, and its sequelae. The major concerns we face today, the group placed as:

— the age imperative: the significance of longevity;
— the child imperative: the impact of poverty;
— the AIDS imperative and drugs: the impact on all of us.

The major issue that must be addressed is for a national health policy that is no longer incremental and specific issue related, but comprehensive.

IV. The Education of the Professions group identified that the language of social-health care remains profession specific and not comprehensive. The group believed that each profession should define its task and functions so that quality collaboration could take place and duplication and turf conflicts avoided. Quality social-health care is truly interprofessional in nature with consultation contributing to sound determinations. Education for consultation, intraprofessional functions, and interdisciplinary care is still faulty and remains a requirement in the curriculum of each of the health care professions.

V. The Research and Evaluation group registered a first concern with the fact that research is used more for its political purposes than for the research consequences themselves. While there was much said about the inherent bias and limited objectivity in much research, the need for information and data is critical for any planning process. A wish for practice enhancement projects was expressed with emphasis on current clinical problems. Such clinical research should be multi-professional in nature. Patient and provider satisfaction with the care delivered were thought to be valued contributions to enhancing service delivery. Also, a major factor missing in current social-health research is the social costs of care. Too little emphasis has been given to the social consequences of disease and the nature of care given in both psychological and economic terms.

Bess Dana synthesizes the papers presented in the workshops and the deliberation of the participants. Mrs. Dana highlights the key points of the "think" pieces and the excellent discussion, quoting liberally from both sources in reflecting on the ongoing struggle between the medical establishment and the outside social community. She helps us not only to understand the language of modern medical care but the range of changes that have taken place and their implications as perceived by the workshop participants. In synthesizing the wide ranging discussions, Mrs. Dana values their professional and interprofessional nature. In citing their perceptions of today's delivery she re-affirms the value of specialization to society's benefit, but underpins the need to "harmonize the efforts" of the specialists "whose differences in knowledge and skills are essential to the identification and solution of social-health problems."

She notes the deep concern for the effects of the influence of government controls and containment initiatives not only on institutions' and providers' behaviors, but also on the social climate of the medically at-risk. She reflects on the participants' wish for changes which guarantee quality care on an equitable and just basis to all Americans. There appears to be rising interest in the health care community for prevention and health maintenance. All agreed that consumers need to be knowledgeable not only for their broad social-health needs but for their own personal health care. Consumers and providers need to be partners in care and in policy determination.

All the clinicians cited the separation of the educational and research communities from the practice world. They faulted these for their lack of preparation in offering comprehensive care of their patients. All cited the need for changes in the academic enterprise to deal with the changing demands on and responsibilities of the health professional. Mrs. Dana notes the differences today from fifteen years ago in the quality of collaboration and in the interaction among the different health care professionals, with the belief that a social-health integration of care is more in evidence today than it was in the past.

The final chapter by Rehr and Rosenberg deals with conclusions and recommendations, in which they restate today's and tomorrow's problems and offer predictions to deal with them.

The planning for a colloquium dealing with a subject of this complexity calls for the contributions of many people. Rehr, Rosenberg, and Dana undertook to spearhead this event and drew on the assistance of the sub-committee for planning. The deliberations on the subject, the hope for extended and in-depth discussions led to the selection of the best keynoters, "think" piece authors, and workshop participants from the field at large. In addition, an event of this magnitude requires organization as well as opportunities for hospitality and socialization. To these ends, we owe so much to Ms. Susan Crimmins, Mrs. Marjorie Pleshette, Mrs. Robert Levinson, Mrs. Marvin Schur, and to the Auxiliary Board members for making the event as successful as it was. For myself, as always, I owe Janice Paneth special tribute for her loving commitment to all the Doris Siegel Colloquia and for extraordinary help in making this fifth event and its publication a reality.

Part II

Presentations

Health Care Today and Tomorrow

Dennis O'Leary

It is an honor for me to have the opportunity to participate in this Colloquium and it is a pleasure to be back in New York City and New York State, which may surprise some of you when I mention that New York is one of the Joint Commission's favorite states.

This topic today is also particularly pleasurable to me because it gives me an opportunity to speculate a little bit about our current environment and what all of that means for the future. I am sure many of you have heard speeches on the future before. Those of us in the health care field cannot resist making predictions. People, particularly like myself and Emily Friedman, who will follow me, are even known to be outrageous, but our saving grace as you can well imagine is that we know that most of you will not remember what we say today and will probably attribute to us something totally different in a few weeks.

I would like at the outset to summarize the basic theme of what I am going to say, because I think it will help you put things in the context of the greater detail that I will provide. First of all I think it should be clear, despite all current turbulence in our environment, that health care services will continue to be a high priority of our society. In spite of lots of turbulence, lots of complaints, and lots of grousing, people cherish health in this country and they will continue to want their care to be available and of the highest quality.

Health care in the future will become even more diversified and more specialized than it is today, if that is possible. I think it is possible. This diversification, this specialization, will require the services of a whole variety of health professionals, many of whom

---

Dennis O'Leary, MD, is President of the Joint Commission on Accreditation of Health Organizations.

are currently identified and providing care. Also, I would suspect that we will see new types of practitioners as health care evolves in the future.

The dark cloud that will hover over us today and tomorrow is the one that reflects that resources are limited. Our resources, which are very much limited today, are so in part because we do not always use them wisely. Indeed, sometimes we waste them, and even misallocate them. We are paying the price today and we will have to rethink health care to fit into the future fiscal constraints.

Tomorrow's health care will belong to teams of providers, not individuals. The reason is clear. Those of us who provide health care, particularly those who are within health care organizations, are coming to understand that the very center of what we do is called the "patient"—the patient as a whole being. We can no longer fragment the patient in the delivery of service. We have learned that the patient is best served if he or she is kept whole, intact, and his/her care is comprehensive and coordinated. To achieve those goals a group of people need to work together. The winning teams tomorrow will have to demonstrate their quality and to provide value to the people who purchase that care. That is the sum and substance of my theme this afternoon. If any of you are given to late afternoon naps you may indulge yourself now as I go to recap some of this.

We may wonder at times how we got to where we are and where it is we are going, but it is really not a mystery. Where we are derives in a very real sense from some social values that we, to various extent, all hold dear. I am not a sociologist, so this may sound a little bit naive, but I think you'll know what I am talking about. We are first of all an affluent society, actually *the* affluent society. We think of ourselves that way. We can afford whatever it is we need and we differ, therefore, from other societies and nations around the world. Indeed, it has only been in this decade with some of the economic problems that we have faced, including a recession, that there has been some realization, not deep, but some realization that our resources are finite. Of course, in health care the finiteness of our resource has become a little bit more brutally clear. With all said and done, we spend immense sums of money on health care and in a broad sense, we are not suffering that much.

Secondly, we are a consumption-oriented society. We consume all kinds of things at an extraordinary clip. It is almost a social pastime for many in this country, and we should not be stunned or astounded, that we, therefore, consume a lot of health care, because that is something that we think is very important. Thirdly, this is only in part tongue in cheek, we are almost uniquely in this world preoccupied with our bodies. This society has an extraordinary somatic orientation that is very clearly central to health care, but extends well beyond that. Indeed, the fads that revolve around exercise programs, jogging, what have you, have led to the creation of whole new medical specialties — like sport medicine. And finally, we are a society that very clearly values quality of life and we translate that to mean available health care. A great deal of the care that is delivered is for the purpose of improving quality of life. Yes, we have a fragmented health care system, and there are certainly inequities within that system, but there are no waiting queues for care. We do not render care based upon what value we as a society will get out of that investment. We invest in quality for the sake of quality.

Those values have been around for a long time and we should not be surprised that for the past two or three decades we have been, in a sense, acting out our commitment to those values. We come from a time period, let's say three decades ago, when you solved problems generally by throwing money at them. We have done that to support health care. Our investments in research, in health care facilities, particularly hospitals, in person power, and finally in patient care, have been outstanding. The research enterprise in this country is large. We have developed new procedures, new techniques, new drugs, and we have translated our research findings into health care delivery at a fairly rapid rate. We have built hospitals in particular, but other health related facilities also, at a staggering clip largely aided by the Hill-Burton Act, which is now history. However, the obligations incurred under that Act are not history, billions of dollars lay there. In regard to health care professionals, a physician shortage was declared by Washington about two decades ago. There was not a lot of data to back up this finding, but it was declared and the government proceeded to create a variety of incentives to repair that problem. And what happened subsequently was mind-blowing to many people, because in essence, we doubled the annual output of our medical schools in less than ten years. Today we are said to have a physician surplus, but the spigot is still on. What are we going to do with all these physicians into the future is not entirely clear, but they certainly will be with us. And of course, we have invested billions of dollars in patient care through the entitlement programs and though these do not work well, they are making possible the delivery of care that might not otherwise have been possible. We may look back and wonder about the wisdom of those investments or wonder whether we might have gotten a greater yield for the dollars that we have invested, but no one is turning off the flow. The investment, in fact, goes up every year, I think, as a fundamental reflection of the things that we as a society believe in. That doesn't mean that people haven't gotten nervous and concerned along the way.

The era of the 1970s in particular, was one of great anxieties, but perhaps not so much in health care. Amongst economists, and payers, and government, the anxieties rose as they watched the portion of the Gross National Product committed to health care rise steadily and it still has not quite leveled off. We do not, most of us simple people, really grasp what the Gross National Product means, but simply put we are told it means that we are buying health care in lieu of other things in our daily lives. It became apparent as well in the 1970s that our reimbursement system encouraged utilization and created few incentives for prudent utilization. It was true in institutional-based care, i.e., hospitals, and certainly it was true in the manner in which we have paid physicians. Those incentives in no small measure are responsible for the rather explosive escalation of health care costs throughout that period of time which amazingly exceeded inflation — which itself was at double digit levels.

We had a technology explosion in the 1970s, too, that was part of the imperative to translate research into health services delivery, and we certainly did that. We did that so quickly that we found ourselves using technology of whose worth we were not quite sure. But who cared, because somebody was going to pay for it. However, we rapidly developed a capacity to deliver care beyond our ability to pay for it. That was the sobering realization with which we were left as we departed the 1970s. Maybe even more serious was the fact that our technological capabilities rapidly outstripped our ethical sophistication. We not only had the ability to provide the quality of life, we had the ability to take patients beyond into a never-never land with which we dealt with great discomfort, and we are not doing all that much better right now.

If we, in health care, had been a little bit more concerned about some of the things that were happening in the 1970s, we might not be where we are today. But on the other hand, we might well be there, whatever one's retrospectoscope says. Very clearly the 1980s have been the years of change. Sooner or later the health care cost issue was going to come to a head. You cannot keep priming the pump indefinitely. What happened was interesting. I am not a Washington, DC native, but I lived there 18 years and the stuff gets under your skin a little bit. This was a classic situation of perception driving policy. It was as if the politicians woke up one morning and said, "there are an awful lot of doctors out there, and there are an awful lot of hospitals out there, and there are probably more out there than there are patients to use them." They went on to say "that means that we've got some leverage for the first time." No one really had done any statistical studies about this. They just decided that was the way it was, and that was when the system started to change rapidly and in a dizzying fashion that really has not yet come to a stop.

Now, I am not going to walk through all the changes that you know about, but I'll highlight a couple.

First of all, the government discovered something, which I think I really discovered about five years earlier but didn't tell anybody, and that it was really silly to keep writing reams of regulations which the government did with great art in the 1970s, when all you had to do was simply say "we are not going to pay for it." But they did discover that in the 1980s, and of course, that is very much a part of health policy in Washington right now. The government also discovered that as a practical course that it would ultimately be best served by attempting to limit its financial risk, and to shift that risk on to other people. This is a course which might not be one that we applaud. The government is certainly not quite where it would like to be. The ideal world for government, as it sees it, would be a capitated system where it lays out its financial commitment up front. It then says to everyone "that is all there is, and you providers or you insurers, or you whoever, are now in the barrel, and if you run out of money, that's too bad, and if you don't run out of money, well God Bless you." Of course, the problem is we usually run out of money.

Out of this mindset, also, arose the concept of competition. The purchasers realized that if government now had all this leverage against an overbedded, and over physician supplied system, well they had some leverage too. Purchasers had been buying health care a la carte, e.g., piecemeal all these years, and now were able to say it would be awfully nice if somebody could provide us a package of services. In the early 1980s, they said we will shop for everything that we need, e.g., for packages of services, preferably cheap. That idea is still very much with us today. We also, along the line, and not very suddenly, decided to change the incentives in this system. All of a sudden there were incentives to provide less care as opposed to more care. This was symbolized by the health maintenance organization movement, but it has been reflected in a variety of other activities. Competition, that they said would never come to health care, has arrived. Now we have fully recognized that health care does not meet the ideal economist definition of a perfect market place. If you go out in the street lots of competition is going on. A lot of people think that's good. There is, let us remind ourselves, a downside to this equation because when you compete, it would be awfully nice if you are not burdened with providing free care to 37 million uninsured Americans. They interfere with your competitive posture. Someone seems to have forgotten that along the line. I am not going to elaborate on this issue, because Emily is going to talk more about it, but it is, probably one of the saddest downsides of what has happened in this decade.

Finally, this decade has given us marked shifts in where patients are cared for, which has a lot of implications for those who own and operate settings of care, more particularly those who provide services. The incentives are all over the place to move care outside of the hospitals. The technology makes the delivery of the services possible. Increasingly competent practitioners can provide services in new settings. There are dollar incentives to move the care out of hospitals. This is absolutely happening and I think that we are more at the beginning of this curve than we are at the end of it.

Those are comments on the background, but for my point of view the big thing that happened in this decade, and I would admit that I bring some bias to this discussion, is that quality of care finally became a real issue, a real public policy issue in this country. Not a big surprise, perhaps except to some of us who have been trying to make quality of care an issue for the previous 20 years and thought that would never happen. But it happened for very logical reasons. If you keep turning the system upside down and turn it upside down again, pretty soon somebody is going to get nervous about the impact of all these changes upon quality care, and of course that did happen.

Today if you are a provider of health care either as an organization or an individual, a lot of people are interested in what you are doing and how well you are doing it. This is the era of public accountability. Perhaps New Yorkers understand that better than anyone else. One is providing care in a goldfish bowl and it is going to be that way for a long time to come. We also have professional liability problems that we are attempting to address. There are a lot of reasons for this professional liability crisis of which we are in the midst. One of the principal causes of this is malpractice. I think we have to recognize that malpractice surfaces the quality issue again, as well as the obvious need to pay attention to what you are doing, because some of what is being done is dangerous to patients. Every now and then somebody has a misadventure, that is readily translated into a seven or eight figure settlement. Competition itself has become linked to the quality issue. This is a young competitive market, and we should not be surprised that it has been driven at the outset by price. But the price alone rarely serves as a sole basis for segregating a market. People will look for something more substantial to achieve that and I think there is a fairly uniform consensus now that quality of care is going to be the basis upon which the future market will separate itself. That, of course, makes the assumption that people will have an ability to prove or to demonstrate, not only to their own satisfaction, but the satisfaction of others that they are really providing high quality care. I think that assumption in fact is real, not a small challenge, but it is a valid assumption. In this environment, interestingly, we now are faced and have been over the past few years, with compelling, strident demands for more sophisticated systems to measure and monitor the quality of care. Government is doing so because government, of course, is the one who changed the system and is now worried whether there were really some quality implications resulting from all these changes. Now, I'd like to tell you that government is altruistic, but it is really not so altruistic. It is worried about being blamed for all the changes. Good measuring systems, those that monitor care, give you a vehicle for blaming someone else eventually.

We also have severe pressures amongst purchasers of care who, of course, are feeling the continued bite of rising health care cost. That is a serious issue. If you are a purchaser, employers most often, whose health care costs are translated into the cost of products and services, which then do not compete as well in the international market place, you have serious concern about employee health care benefits. It is a dollars and cents issue that tracks itself back to appropriateness of care perhaps more than to quality. However, one answer to that problem is to direct the employees to low cost, and, hopefully, good providers. Unfortunately, that linkage is not yet clear. At this time, a lot of American businesses are in the process of doing fairly detailed profiles of hospitals, physicians, and other kinds of practitioners. But, all that activity will do is give them an utilization and cost profile, not the essentials of quality care. If one goes the preferred provider pathway (PPO), and tells your employees that they must go to a given provider, and the employee having gone to this provider has a little misadventure you know what is going to happen. The legal suit will start with the provider, but it will make its way back to the employer. This is not a theoretical consideration. It is happening already, and the effect is a sort of paralysis among the purchasers of care. Obviously what they need is to get a handle on some quantitative data, a firm handle on quality care, so that they can direct their employees more safely to the good providers. So clearly, there is pressure in that sector, as well. There are a number of organizations, including my own organization, that are now deeply invested in developing these new methods for measuring and monitoring quality. I can tell you this is a highly doable kind of task, but it is also highly complex. If anybody is looking for a deliverable solution by Monday, forget it. We are not going to have that solution so soon. We will have pieces of it, like data profiles, but that is not what quality evaluation is all about.

Ultimately, we in health care will face a mandate for self-examination. You are hearing some of that from your friendly department of health. It is just beginning. None of us comes by self-examination naturally or comfortably. Let us all admit that. Self-examination is a very good idea for someone else to do. But self-examination we will need to have, otherwise we will be subject to a variety of examinations, not all of which will be fairly based. That is also a reality, not theory.

And so the challenge for today for providers, individuals, and organizations, and for the future, the way it is going to be, is to look at what we do, understand what we do, fix our problems, and capitalize on opportunities to do better tomorrow what we are already doing reasonably well today. What all this means is looking at patient care and its management. These are two things we have studiously stayed away from all these decades. In order to do this, we will need data and information. In the future, quality of care will be data based or data driven quality assurance. Whether it turns out based on work that JCAHO has done and work that others are doing, there is no problem identifying performance, monitors, or indicators, whatever you would like to call them. They are things that are reasonably related to the quality of care delivered and can be measured. In these systems the data are not an end in themselves — a trap into which the Health Care Financing Administration and others have already fallen. No one will deny the data become an extremely important vehicle for raising questions about the quality of care at the very least, and will probably point one in the direction of problems that are subject to resolution. A lot of people are going to be interested in performance information in the future. This interest will become a centerpiece of our health care lives. This is not an unhappy occurrence if you happen to be a patient. Wouldn't you like to be cared for in an environment where everybody cared about providing quality care, where people felt good about finding problems or finding opportunities to improve performance all built around you, the patient? That kind of culture change is what we are really talking about. I think it should provide some reassurance to government. It would give purchasers an ability to ask the right kinds of questions and to meet the consumer's demand, which is value for their dollar. They don't expect care to be cheap, but they do want value for their dollar. Some people look at the complexities of these new evaluation systems as though they are overwhelming. But I can tell you today, that if I were a purchaser of care, I have got my questions all ready for the provider. I would ask:

— "Do you have a quality assurance plan? I'd like to see it."
— "What do you monitor here?"
— "What kind of data, performance data do you look at?"
— "Do you have some I could see?"
— "What do these data mean to you?"
— "How do you use them?"
— "What kind of problems or issues did the data raise?"
— "What did you do about them?"
— "When you did something about them, did that improve things?"
— "Can I know a few changes you have introduced?"

A quality organization will be one in a position to answer these questions. There is a fundamental recognition that the objective of what we are about is not perfection. We will not achieve perfection. Let us forget that. What we are trying to achieve is an atmosphere, a cultural environment in which the premium is on continuous improvement in performance. We need to keep trying to do better tomorrow what we already are doing reasonably well today.

You should glean a little bit from what I have said, that tomorrow is not about individuals; it is not about pieces of turf; it is not about fragmentation. If you look at the truly successful health care organizations around the country today, these are integrated and internally coordinated. You can hardly tell these players apart because they all sing from the same hymnal. They get their jobs done by working together. The jobs inside organizations today are so complex, you cannot get a job done all by yourself, and that is true whether you are looking at an organization from a government's standpoint, a management's standpoint, or if you are trying to provide care to the patient. You are going to need teams of people who work together, who individually respect each other's competence and skills, and who know that everybody on the team brings something to bear that is going to be of value to the patient. And naturally if you want to be crass about that, you can sell it, because that is what people want. That is what they will ultimately buy. Now, that doesn't mean that if you are a rugged individualist that you are going to have an impossible time tomorrow. There will still be niches out there for the individualist. However, everyone should bear in mind whether they are the individual practitioner or part of a team, that it is performance that is going to count tomorrow. It will be nice to have all those certificates on the wall, saying you graduated from such and such, or you have such and such special training, or you are certified by such and such special society, but that is not going to count as much tomorrow. With a data based quality assurance system, people are going to want to know what you do, and how well you do it. Our titles and certificates will come to mean less. Speaking from a physician's perspective, we have watched a variety of practitioners develop competencies. People will constantly, I think, keep trying to upgrade themselves. In my view if they are demonstratably good at that, so be it. Those people who are working their way up the ladder in terms of gaining a broader involvement in the system must be mindful of those people who are coming up behind them. We see that happening in various professional fields. However, ultimately, the consumer will pass judgment. The consumer of health care is neither naive nor stupid. You will see his/her judgment acted out in a variety of ways. Ultimately, it will be quality that is going to pay off. Consumers do know something about that. Some people are uncomfortable with consumer involvement in health care determinations. I have many colleagues who wring their hands anxiously about the present and the future, but happily many more colleagues see some opportunities in this environment, opportunities to do a better job. Despite competition and turbulence and other problems in our environment, there will always be room for people who provide a needed service done very well. Patients will always exist. People need health care, and let's remember that it is those people who matter. If they weren't here then we wouldn't be here. But they are here and we need to be here for them in a spectacular fashion.

Thank you.

Patients as Partners:
The Changing Health Care Environment

Emily Friedman

I have always an ambivalent reaction when I am asked to talk about forces that will influence the future. This is because predictions tend to provoke strange reactions. One popular approach is to base one's entire strategic plan on what others say will happen, which can be an efficient way to commit professional suicide. Or one can embrace one little piece of a prediction — usually a piece that is pleasing because it consists of exactly what we want to hear — and can put all his or her marbles in that thin little basket. That can be a visionary thing to do, but it does go against the odds. As Peter Drucker has said, "Miracles are great, but they are so damned unpredictable." Or one can ignore all the predictions and do what instinct suggests, which also has merit.

What I think is the best reaction, however, is to consider the part of the prediction that is the most frightening, and try to think in terms of what would be required of you if it came true. This is in keeping with the wonderful observation by E. W. Howe that a "good scare is worth more than good advice."

Confronting the unwanted event is more difficult, of course, because it requires a recognition that the future may not be what we want it to be. On the other hand, it helps one learn to deal with the undesired and the unexpected. That is a skill well worth nurturing, for what wasn't supposed to be, but happened anyway, has become a common event of our times. Knowledge of that uncomfortable fact can breed vision and creativity in those who take the future seriously.

Emily Friedman is contributing Editor for *Hospitals, Medical World News, Healthcare Forum Journal,* and *Health Business*.

As Rudyard Kipling observed in his poem, "The Benefactors":

Ah! What avails the classic bent
And what the cultured word,
Against the undoctored incident
That actually occurred?

And what is Art whereto we press
Through paint and prose and rhyme —
When Nature in her nakedness
Defeats us every time?

It is not learning, grace, nor gear
Nor easy meat and drink,
But bitter pinch of pain and fear
That makes creation think.

The other quality that I think is most helpful in trying to respond to the forces of change is a willingness to let go of a long-cherished American tradition: our self-defeating habit of insisting that there is only one answer to a problem, one reason for a situation, and one force at work in a process.

The forces that are at work like termites in health care's walls are a good deal more complex than we would like. One thing that makes them so, of course, is the interminable snake dance that constitutes our health policy process. Its most salient rule is two steps forward, one step back. Wilbur Cohen, author of the law that brought Medicaid and Medicare into being, used to say that when an issue flowers, American legislators will pass any sort of dumb measure to address it, and then spend the rest of their lives tinkering with it. Thus there is a slight twist in the policy snake dance, which is that most politicians can be counted on to step out of the line from time to time and do a little mambo on the side.

But, despite appearances, politicians do not operate in a vacuum. Every once in a while, usually every two, four, or six years, they have to produce a show of accountability. What usually governs that accountability are the larger forces — over which they often have little control — that have become powerful enough to move the common man and woman. And public interest will, in time, move the politician, unless an extraordinarily effective lobby intervenes, which has been true in the case of sensitive issues like handgun control and abortion. With those relatively few exceptions, social forces cause political action, sooner or later.

In terms of these larger, broader trends, I think five sets of forces, each the product of a profound conflict, are moving to shape 21st century health care. Each is an example of dynamic tension: whichever force proves more powerful when the music stops will have a great influence on our system and the people who use it.

The first, and most politically powerful, conflict is the need for health care versus access to health care. A growing imbalance here has heated up the issue. For a long time, need and access were in *relative* balance — and I emphasize *relative* — because access has always been a problem in this country. But now we are headed for a fall.

The number of people with no public or private coverage for their health care costs has mushroomed, to 37 million, a 38 percent increase over the 1977 figure.[1] Hospitals, which for a long time defused the problem by providing uncompensated care, have not been able to keep up as the number of uninsured exploded, payment policy changed, and hospital philosophies, in many cases, hardened.

Today, the majority of the uninsured have compromised on nonexistent access to health care except when they are in extremis. As social work professionals know far too well, hospitals will usually (not always, but usually) rush in at the last moment like the cavalry and pull these patients back from the grave, but that hardly serves as a solution. It doesn't produce very good outcomes, and it is terribly expensive.

We must understand what's going on here. If Americans did not think there is a basic right to health care, they would let hospitals and physicians refuse to treat the dying uninsured and let them expire on the steps in front of them. But we have instead instituted statutory, regulatory, civil, and moral guarantees that one at least should get care if one is dying or having a baby.

So access for the uninsured is often a matter of timing. What they do *not* have access to are things like primary care, prenatal care, well-baby care, screening for cancer and other diseases, immunization, and other interventions. This has its effects. Our infant mortality rate of 10.4 deaths per 1,000 births, places us in 19th place—just about dead last—among developed nations. Our rate for nonwhite infants places us behind nations such as Bulgaria and Cuba.[2] Between eight and 15 American mothers die for every 100,000 births, and the rate for black women is three and a half times that.[3-4] That puts us behind most developed countries and many Third World countries.

Often, however, members of the mainstream middle class, including many hospitals and physicians, do not see this issue as touching them. They are wrong: this hole in our collective heart is also a hole in our collective head, for medical indigence affects us all. In September 1988, a Chicago Vietnam veteran who was known to be mentally ill went for a walk with his gun (which he owned legally, in my retrograde state) and killed four people, including a woman police officer who was the mother of four children, the owners of an auto parts store, and a maintenance man at a school. Much of the carnage took place at a school for disturbed children; we do not yet know what toll may have been taken on them. All the people who were killed were employed and middle class. The uninsured are not members of some other species whose problems do not touch us.

The uninsured are also often the targets of precedents that will come back to haunt us—precedents we allowed to be set because we did not see any connections between them and our own situations. Health insurers have won the battle, except in California, to test individual applicants for health insurance for antibodies to human immunodeficiency virus (HIV), which causes acquired immune deficiency syndrome (AIDS). One recent study found that life insurance firms (health insurers will likely follow) are testing blood pulled for HIV testing for other conditions, like drugs and diabetes.[5] Both Prudential and Travelers report that they are rejecting more applicants now than a few years ago.[5] Wisconsin insurers have proposed that they be allowed to test all members of any applicant group of 25 workers or less, and choose which of them they will insure.[6] On a personal note, I had a terrible time trying to get an individual policy to cover me while I was out of state for a year. I work out every morning, don't cook with salt, don't drink hard liquor, don't use drugs, don't even drink coffee—and came within 48 hours of being uninsured.

Indeed, medical indigence is already a fact of life for many in the working class, and is beginning to eat into the middle class. I recently asked a commercial insurance representative where he thought it all would end, given that we will soon be able to test for latent alcoholism, hypertension, and predisposition to cancer. He responded, laughing, that the insurers couldn't screen everyone out, or "we'd underwrite ourselves right out of business." I wasn't laughing. The commercial insurers in this country have started down a slippery slope, and I don't think either they or the rest of us know at what point they are planning to stop—and whether they will be able to stop when they want to.

Add to this dilemma the well-documented decline and fall of Medicaid, which now covers less than half of those with income below the poverty line, the growth in that poverty population, and the overcrowding of our urban public hospitals.[7-9] Stir in the demographic juggernaut, which just keeps chugging along. The baby boomers are turning 40 at the rate of 9,300 a day, and will continue to do so for another 15 years. There are already more people over 65 than there are teenagers. Older Americans use more health services than do younger Americans (something we have lately taken to blaming them for, in this age of the Yuppie and unbridled personal greed). The demographics are such that even if we didn't extend coverage to one more person, and if health care capital expenditures froze, we would still add millions of dollars to the health care bill every week.

The fact is—like it or not—that the collapse of Medicaid, the eroding availability of commercial insurance, the precarious finances of Blue Cross and Blue Shield (which lost $1.9 billion last year), the aging of the population, and skyrocketing health care costs are combining to force this country into designing and implementing some sort of universal entitlement. I believe, based on the comments of politicians, that it will happen soon—certainly by the end of the century—regardless of who is president at the time the legislation is passed.

For the fact is that Congress will be running the country for the next few years. And Congress is extremely interested in addressing this issue. Numerous recent trade press reports quote key congressional leaders as saying that the elderly got the catastrophic package, and now it's time to do something about the medically indigent. The people being quoted include Republicans and Democrats, liberals and conservatives. They realize what too few providers have realized: that the infrastructure of the health care system and state and local finances is grievously threatened by the overwhelming burden of caring (and not caring) for the uninsured. Already, several states have moved on this issue: not only Massachusetts, but also Hawaii, Oregon, Vermont, Pennsylvania, Michigan, and others. There are even rumblings in conservative spots like Missouri and California. Legislation sponsored by Senator Edward Kennedy (D-MA) and Representative Henry Waxman (D-CA), which would require employers to cover all full-time employees and some part-time employees, has garnered the support of strange bedfellows like American Airlines, Chrysler Corporation, the Catholic Health Association, the American Hospital Association, and Karl Bays, chairman of the board of IC Industries in Chicago. A poll by *Hospitals* magazine found that 75 percent of Americans support mandatory employee health insurance.[10] The writing is on the wall.

Furthermore, every politician I have heard speak about this issue talks about getting two things done at once: universal coverage and health care system reform. The process of solving medical indigence is going to be systemic. It will not consist solely of expanding Medicaid, or increasing payments to obstetricians, or subsidizing hospitals that provide a lot of indigent care. It's going to go deeper than that.

Need for personnel versus availability of personnel, the second set of forces involves the human factor. As it stands now, we have a huge health care sector with high personnel demands, and a health care work force that is increasingly mismatched to those demands.

Demographics figure here as well. The baby boom has been fairly efficiently swallowed by the giant maw of American employment, which burped a little but employed most of them — not always in the world's greatest jobs, but in jobs nonetheless. Now the baby bust is upon us. And the flip side of the growing shortage of young workers is that health care will have to compete for them with other employment sectors that may be more attractive.

The second demographic factor is the emergence of women as a political and social power. The shortage of hospital nurses is a key illustration of that; 78.6 percent of U.S. hospitals have nursing shortages, with more than half reporting vacancies of 10 percent or more.[11]

The common wisdom is that nurses are underpaid, which they are, and that the demand for nursing has increased, which it has, and that accounts for the nursing shortage. This scenario assumes that more money and better utilization of nurses will solve the problem. But two other factors are involved here that are harder to crack — and are emblematic of a larger issue in health care employment. First, health care staffing was predicated — *structured* — on a belief that most women had only the choice of teaching, nursing, or staying home and being parents. Is it, therefore, not surprising that health care has long been dominated by women workers; the health care work force is about 80 percent female.[12] But today, women can be nuclear physicists, politicians, and — most telling — physicians. Of the graduating medical school class of 1988, 32.8 percent were women.[13] Nursing now must compete with other attractive options (and I think nursing remains a very attractive option), both within and outside health care. And many of those professions pay better and provide more power to women.

Also, despite the disproportionate role women play in the provision of health care, they have often been relatively powerless, ignored, or even abused. A recent survey of nurses about what they considered their toughest moral dilemmas on the job disclosed the following five most common complaints: "no code" orders; performance of unnecessary tests or treatments for profit or to protect from malpractice; lying to or withholding information from patients; incompetence or inadequate treatment by physicians; and performance of tests without informed consent or with no consent.[14] Even a cursory examination of that list reveals that these nurses are now complaining about physician behavior. And in an era of physician oversupply and nurse undersupply, the forces of change are with the nurses. I think the forces of change will be with women in many other health care professions as well. For example, today most physicians involved in managed care must seek the permission of a female nurse in order to hospitalize a patient.

Yet while all this demographic change is surfacing, the top layer of health care management and governance remains overwhelmingly male and white. Of active affiliates of the American College of Healthcare Executives, only 9.8 percent are lay women hospital administrators; of 4,500 hospital CEO's, only 187 are lay women.[15] The image that comes to mind is what I call the "plantation model." Health care is a largely female, increasingly nonwhite work force presided over by a thin, white male layer at the top. This is anachronistic in a world where most of the available new workers are going to be female and often Asian, Black, and Hispanic.[16]

Medicine is giving us a preview of the type of change the new demographics are provoking. In the 1960s, Lyndon Johnson and Congress moved to increase the then-tight U.S. supply of physicians. By 1980, the Graduate Medical Education Advisory Committee issued a report saying that the United States was about to be knee-deep in doctors. So we moved to cut the rate of increase in the supply. Now there is a debate about whether the aging population, AIDS, and other trends might increase need for care to the point that it might overtax the existing physician supply. That fight will go on and on, for the stakes are sky-high for medical schools, teaching hospitals, medically underserved areas, cost control proponents, and other interests.

But this much we know is true: We produce too many specialists in relation to primary care physicians, who are already in short supply in some areas.[17] Physicians swarm in certain places, mostly urban and suburban, but many areas of the United States are chronically underserved or unserved by physicians. Even in the San Francisco Bay Area, a recent report found that although the physician-to-patient ratio in the city is at most 160:1, in one low-income area the ratio was 1 physician for 8,300 patients.[18]

Overall physician income is still rising—it averaged $119,500 in 1986, a 6.5 percent increase over 1985; but for young physicians, it is not rising much.[19] And because of different attitudes and the influx of young women into the profession, younger physicians are seeking group practice and salaried or contract employment in un-precedented numbers.

All this is breeding new phenomena. One is that the traditional closing of ranks among physicians is getting less close all the time. There are physicians who don't have enough work, and there is a growing fear on the part of consumers that those physicians may start generating unnecessary work. Physicians are starting to be less than collegial with each other and with other professionals—nurse practitioners, physician's assistants, chiropractors, and so on—who seek to increase even further what some of us cynically refer to as the patient shortage (which, as more and more people become unin-sured, will only become more acute).

The effect of the changes that are shaking medicine's socks, for better or worse, cannot be overestimated. We are going to witness the rise in prestige and income of heretofore slighted specialties like geriatrics, rehabilitation medicine, family practice, and psychiatry, because they are in tune with what much future health care need will be. We will see what has been the unimaginable: a compromise of the top-of-the-heap position held by surgery and other procedural specialties, a process that will be accelerated when Medicare moves to a relative value scale (which I don't think it will do). As physi-cians fall to quarreling over whose specialty is more cognitive and deserves what rate of reimbursement, the traditional pecking order will be shaken up. There will be a redistribution of income among specialties, and a redistribution of power between medicine and nursing. This, in and of itself, is a revolution.

Overall, health care will have a work force that is in a much better bargaining position, that is redefining its work and aspira-tions, and that is demographically radically different from the work force of the past.

Perceived quality versus real quality; how the quality of health care will be defined underlies the third big collision of forces. This is another extremely high-stakes game. The major weapon that will swing the balance is the quantification of quality—the growing use of data collection and analysis to determine the quality of care.

For too many years, health care providers defined quality in the way described by William Guy, former president of Blue Cross of

California: "What *I* do is quality; what *you* do is shlock." Now, we are starting, thanks to the unholy combination of eager health services researchers, cost-conscious payers, and cynical regulators, to draw a bead on what constitutes quality.

Providers defined quality on the basis of four dubious principles. First, the Cartesian principle, as in "I think, therefore I am": "Because I provide American health care, it must be good, because American health care is the best in the world." Second was "the more, the better"; this is the American way. Third, "quality equals money." The more you pay the better the care. Fourth, "health care is an art that defies quantification." Providers, when challenged, could prove none of these claims. Now they have the choice of either participating in radical change, or being run over by an idea whose time has come with a vengeance. Many providers— especially physicians, to their credit—have dabbled a toe in these new waters, but time pressure is forcing more major commitments.

What is happening is actually relatively simple. Information about how health care works is being collected and analyzed, and the results are being made public, almost always with the approval of consumer groups, and often with the active participation of consumer groups. Quality and data are no longer the exclusive realm of the inner sanctum of the quality review committees; now they are on the front page of the *Times*. Just to mention a few examples:

- The United States caesarean section rate of 24.4 percent, highest in the world, is indefensible on clinical grounds.[20] More caesareans are performed on women with private insurance than on women with Medicaid or no insurance, which really raises questions.[20] Angry insurers and angrier female consumers are starting to act.
- Several big payers, like Blue Cross and Blue Shield of Illinois and Foundation Health Plan in California, now pay less for caesareans than they used to. Foundation Health Plan pays more for a vaginal birth after a caesarean than it does for a caesarean; the Illinois Blues no longer pay a differential for a ceasarean.[20] The Caesarean Prevention Movement, based in Syracuse, has dozens of chapters. Powerful women's health

care consumer groups are here to stay; *Our Bodies, Ourselves* remains a best seller. And women are increasingly powerful in health care; they represent 60 percent of acute care patients, 80 percent of nursing home patients, 90 percent of nursing home patients over 85. And their influence will grow as the population ages, because women live longer than do men, and thus will represent an ever-larger percentage of the population.

- A 1988 study found that lung cancer patients with private health insurance (including Medicare beneficiaries with private supplemental coverage) are more likely to receive surgery, chemotherapy, and radiation therapy than are people who do not have private health insurance (including Medicare clients without private supplemental coverage).[21] We have always believed that once a person enters the health care system (however difficult that is for the uninsured and underinsured), he or she is treated like anyone else, no matter what his or her coverage; that is evidently not the case.

- Questions are being raised about the proliferation of several surgical procedures, including coronary artery bypass graft, carotid endarterectomy, transurethral prostatectomy, and others, given that little research has been done to indicate when they should be performed and what their benefits are.[22-25] This is a natural consequence of the pioneering work of John Wennberg, MD, and his colleagues who found that the rates at which patients are admitted to hospitals, for the same conditions, vary by as much as 1,000 percent.[26]

The quantification of quality will overwhelm provider paternalism, patient ignorance, payer indifference, and the pervasive role of malpractice as an excuse for everything and the solution for all disputes over quality. We will either be able to demonstrate the quality of what is done, through outcomes, or we won't be in business.

The second hottest topic in health care comes into play here. That is what Larry Gage of the National Association of Public Hospitals calls "the 'R' word: rationing. There is a rampant terror in the United States that we will have to ration health care — as though our overflowing public hospitals, payers' refusal to cover the costs of tissue plasminogen activator (TPA) and other drugs, and horrendous infant mortality rate were not silent witness of just how much we already do so.

The question is, as coverage is extended to everyone, on what basis will we ration? We won't be able to do it by restricting access through ability to pay, as we do now. I hope that we will instead ration care on the basis of quality, appropriateness, and effectiveness. Let us seek to do what works best first. Let us set priorities that are clinical first and economic second. We are among a very few developed nations that do not have national health care priorities. Indeed, we have virtually no national health policy at all. I think the new emphasis on quality and outcomes may lead us into a saner and more humane stance. As Winston Churchill said, in my favorite of his many wonderful statements, "Americans can always be counted on to do the right thing—once they have exhausted every possible alternative."

Provider control over health care versus nonprovider control; the fourth balancing act is in some ways the most frightening. It is the question of who is going to control health care: the people who provide it, or the people who pay for it. The role of the patient in this regard will grow markedly in any case, but because of the information monopoly held by providers, patients will never be the masters.

Providers ran the decision-making show for a long time. Now payers have grabbed a good bit of that power. It's a serious situation, because the bad guys have three powerful weapons. First, many Americans resent physicians because their incomes are so high. Second, health care providers, individual and institutional, have more professional freedom than most Americans. Third, health care costs an enormous amount of money, and reducing provider's take, rather than patients' coverage, is very attractive to resentful nonproviders.

What the denouncement will be on this issue is going to be a very, very close call. I do not know if providers can hang onto the territory they have, let alone regain what has been lost to payers. I'm not as worried about territory lost to patients, much of which should have been theirs all along. I do know that I am not thrilled at the prospect of some actuary at Travelers Insurance deciding whether I am worthy of surgery. I cringe at the thought of the Health Care Financing Administration deciding on a fiscal basis whether I will have access to care that will keep me alive, especially as I age in a society that increasingly — and idiotically — seeks to disenfranchise the elderly.

If providers — and I consider everyone who works in or with a health care organization to be a provider — want to retain control of their work, their best chance is to form a sincere partnership with patients and the public, by providing moral leadership on these other issues. And they must work together, rather than quarreling over scraps. As David Kinzer of the Harvard School of Public Health has said, "the strongest ethical position a health care organization can take is to support the ethical commitments of its clinical professionals."

Providers must also abandon paternalism and inflexibility. Health care leaders have long embraced change — but only change that was convenient and easy to take, like broadening health insurance and the unquestioning embrace of new technology. They have been almost stridently resistant to less comfortable change. And they are paying a heavy price for that resistance. But as Pearl Buck once said, "Every great mistake has a halfway moment, a split second when it can be recalled and perhaps remedied." It is not too late.

Public image of providers versus self-image; finally, there is the need to achieve some reasonable relationship between how the public sees health care providers, and how they see themselves. Those two visions have been in imbalance for a long time, but the providers didn't care. When you are being worshipped as gods who can do anything, who cares if the image is inaccurate?

Then came consumerism, the women's movement, anti-institutionalism, taxpayer revolts, and the post-industrial society. All of a sudden physicians are crooks, hospitals don't deserve their tax exemptions, hospital nursing is listed in surveys as one of the worst jobs in the country, patients are suing physicians, medical self-help books become best-sellers as patients seek to protect themselves from the health care system, and an explosion in public questioning of provider morality produces the health care ethics revolution. This sort of thing could make a body feel insecure.

Unfortunately or fortunately, this situation will prevail for some time to come, because the United States, as a nation, is going through a delayed adolescence, and we are questioning everything. We are a very new country, even if we are an old democracy, and we don't have it all down yet. As my friend Simon, an Englishman, says, "The British think a hundred miles is a long way; Americans think a hundred years is a long time."

But out of all this will come the most needed balance of all: a health care system tied far more closely to its patients than it has ever been. A major impetus will be the ongoing process of health care ethics. It is extremely painful to seek answers to questions of care (or non-care) of the dying; prolongation of the lives of fragile, doomed newborns; euthanasia; institutional survival versus community need; confidentiality of sensitive or dangerous information; meaningful informed consent; and how patients and providers can better relate to and trust each other.

But these agonies are healthy. They are producing something that has been in too-short supply in health care: individual and institutional introspection. That, in itself, is a frightening process, for it produces change, and profound change is shattering, whether it is good or bad. The births of babies and the deaths of friends will zonk one out equally effectively.

Nevertheless, hoary old health care, which for so long did an amazingly faithful imitation of the Rock of Gibraltar when it came to being flexible, is undergoing metamorphosis. And new alliances will be born of that. They will be a little weird, I grant you: patients teaming up with clinical caregivers to make decisions about the quality of death; physicians seeking the advice of social workers as the social basis of so much chronic illness is revealed; nurses ordering doctors around; policy makers trying to deal with the problems of people who are included in the system rather than excluded; and the ongoing tension between those who love technology and those who love touch.

Everyone involved will be frightened by some part of this process, but it will still be a good process, and things will come out all right. As H. L. Mencken said, "The good Lord protects dogs, children, drunks, and the United States of America." And as this all unfolds, remember that you will not be alone in going down these new roads. Many of us will be there with you, in the spirit of the inspiring telegram once sent to a college football coach by a faithful alumnus before a big game: "Remember, Coach, we're all behind you—win or tie."

REFERENCES

1. Short, P., et al., *Uninsured Americans: A 1987 Profile*, Rockville, MD, National Center for Health Services Research and Health Care Technology Assessment, 1988. (Data from the 1987 National Medical Expenditures Survey.)

2. Rochat, R., et al., "Maternal Mortality in the United States: Report From the Maternal Mortality Collaborative," *Obstetrics and Gynecology*, 72(1):91-97, July 1988.

3. Children's Defense Fund, *The Health of America's Children: Maternal and Child Health Data Book, 1988*, Washington, DC, The Fund, 1988.

4. Gold, R.B., et al., "Paying for Maternity Care in the United States," *Family Planning Perspectives*, 19(5):190-206, September/October 1987.

5. "Insurers Using AIDS Test to Check for Other Ills," *Blue Cross and Blue Shield Media Digest*, No. 29, July 25, 1988.

6. Mader, M., "The AIDS Concern: Insurance for the Uninsurable," *The Public Eye*, published by the Center for Public Representation, Madison, WI, 13(4):1-4, Spring 1988.

7. Fackelman, K., "Medicaid: Today and Tomorrow," *Medicine & Health Perspectives*, 42(11):1-4, March 14, 1988.

8. Gage, L., et al., *America's Health Safety Net: A Report on the Situation of Public Hospitals in Our Nation's Metropolitan Areas*, Washington, DC, National Association of Public Hospitals, 1987.

9. Joint Economic Committee of Congress, *The Growth in Poverty: 1979-85*, Washington, DC, 1986. *See also*, "Poverty Edges Up In 1987," *Chicago Tribune*, September 1, 1988, p. 6.

10. Shaffer, M., "Seventy-Five Percent of the Public Supports Mandated Benefits," *Hospitals*, 62(17):110, September 5, 1988.

11. "Nursing Shortage Continues," American Hospital Association press release, May 12, 1988.

12. Butter, I., et al., *Sex and Status: Hierarchies in the Health Workforce*, Washington, DC, American Public Health Association, March 1985.

13. "Briefly This Week," *Medicine & Health*, 42(36) J4, September 12, 1988. *See also*, Friedman, E., "Women MDs: Changing the Ranks of Medicine, *Medical World News*, 29(8):56-68, April 25, 1988.

14. "Moral Distress In Nursing," *Hospital Ethics*, 3(4):1-5, July/August 1987.

15. Weil, P., *A Statistical Profile of Affiliates of the American College of Healthcare Executives*, Chicago, American College of Healthcare Executives, 1987. Plus additional data provided personally by Dr. Weil, 1987.

16. Riche, M., "America's New Workers," *American Demographics*, 10(2):34-41, February 1988.

17. Schroeder, S., "Western European Responses to Physician Oversupply," *JAMA*, 252(3):373-383, July 20, 1984. For an overview of the arguments against predictions of oversupply, *see* Jacobsen, S., and Rimm, A., "The Projected Physician Surplus Reevaluated, *Health Affairs*, 6(2):48-56, Summer 1987.

18. Smith, M., "When Physicians Are In Oversupply, Who Serves the Poor?" Paper presented at the annual meeting of the American Public Health Association, New Orleans, October 1987.

19. "Physicians' Net Income Grows Despite Surge In Expenses," *SMS Report*, 1(4):1-2, November, 1987. *See also*, "Changing Practice Patterns for Young Physicians," *SMS Report*, 2(1):2-4, January 1988.

20. Friedman, E., "Consumer Group Calls Half of the Nation's Cesareans Unnecessary," *Medical World News*, 28(24):70-71, December 28, 1987.

21. Greenberg, E.R., et al., "Social and Economic Factors In Treatment of the Choice of Lung Cancer Treatment," *New England Journal of Medicine*, 318(10):612-617, March 10, 1988.

22. *See*, for example, Graboys, T.B., et al., "Results of a Second Opinion Program for Coronary Artery Bypass Graft Surgery," *JAMA*, 258(12):1611-1614, September 25, 1987; Winslow, C.M., et al., "The Appropriateness of Performing Coronary Artery Bypass Surgery," *JAMA*, 260(4):505-509, July 22/29, 1988; and Mulley, A.G., and Eagle, K., "What Is the Inappropriate Care?" *JAMA*, 260(4):540-541, July 22-29, 1988.

23. *See*, for example, Merrick, N., "Use of Carotid Endarterectomy In Five California Veterans Administration Medical Centers," *JAMA*, 256(18):2566-7, November 14, 1986.

24. Barry, M.J., et al., "Watchful Waiting vs. Immediate Transurethral Resection for Symptomatic Prostatism," *JAMA*, 259(20):3010-3017, May 27, 1988; Fowler, F.J., et al., "Symptom Status and Quality of Life Following Prostatectomy," *JAMA*, 259(20), 3018-3022, May 27, 1988; and Wennberg, J.E., et al., "An Assessment of Prostatectomy for Benign Urinary Tract Obstruction," *JAMA*, 259(20):3027-3030, May 27, 1988.

25. Friedman, E., "Practice Variations: Where Will the Push to Fall In Line End?" *Medical World News*, 27(2): 51-69, January 27, 1986.

26. "Top 25 Most Frequently Performed Surgeries," *Healthweek*, 2(13):23, June 20, 1988.

Part III

The "Think" Pieces
and Participants' Deliberations:
A Synthesis

Reaching for the Social-Health Benefits of Medical Care

Bess Dana

THE CONTEXT

> Real change in the modern age requires not the seizure of power, the revolutionary's dream, but the dispersal of power . . . it must be inspired by a sense of the common good or democracy becomes 'boring, fragile, and weak' in the words of Sir Oscar Chadwick, a historian from Cambridge. (Lewis, 1990)

Viewed from the perspective of the underlying values and principles that inform these excerpts from Flora Lewis' essay, *Needs of Civil Society,* the deliberations of the Fifth Doris Siegel Memorial Colloquium represent the translation of her prescription for reaching the benefits of modernity in civil society into the lingus franca of modern medical care. The keynote papers presented at the opening (plenary) session and replicated in full on the preceding pages provide a glossary for understanding the changing medical care vocabulary; its expression in dollar-driven health care policies and regulations; the application of the principles and practices of modern corporate management to the organizational structure and administration of today's medical centers; the growing adaptation of the techniques developed for the marketing and packaging of commercial products to the marketing and packaging of health and medical care services; the legal and judicial actions that challenge the time-honored privileges of health and health-related professions to

Bess Dana, MSW, is Professor of Community Medicine Emerita, Mount Sinai School of Medicine, City University of New York.

49

assess and monitor the quality of their own performance; the growing role of the multi-media as vehicles for acquainting the consumer with both the benefits and deficits of medical science and encouraging the articulation of the voice of the consumer in health and medical affairs; the concomitant growth in the use of the courts and legislative bodies to protect and promote the consumer's access to medical information and the exercise of his/her rights of choice in decisions affecting the nature and duration of medical treatment.

The workshop proceedings, summarized and interpreted in the body of this report, define the new and changing medical care vocabulary in operational terms: its expression in the on-going efforts to members of the various health and health-related professions and disciplines to reconcile their respective norms and expectations of professional behavior and outcomes with the changing demographic characteristics, norms, and expectations of society. The report that follows is intended to capture the key elements in the process and outcome of a morning devoted to the pursuit of this demanding purpose.

The report is based on: (1) an analysis of the "think process" that introduced the particular subject area addressed by each of the five groups into which the workshop component of the Colloquium was sub-divided: Delivery of Personal Clinical Health Services; Organization and Management of Social-Health Resources; Health Policy, Planning and Regulations; Education of the Health Care Professions; Research and Evaluation; (2) The reporters' minutes of each of these five concurrent sessions; (3) Dr. Rehr's notes from the discussion of the post-colloquium meeting of workshop leaders, recorders, and Colloquium planners.

The participants' first-hand experiences, ideas, and the subjective feelings engendered by their daily exposure to the changing conditions of the health care environment are deeply imbedded in these source materials. The "think" pieces provide a cogent analysis of the factors in the external environment and within the biomedical establishment itself that are implicated in the current struggle between the health care community and the larger social community — local, state, and federal governments, special interest groups, and consumer advocates — for control of health affairs.

The reporters' minutes present persuasive evidence of the power of the interchange of experiences, ideas, and feelings to serve as a catalyst for identifying areas of common concern and to break down the barriers that have continued to limit the scope, effectiveness, and professional rewards of interprofessional collaboration.

Dr. Rehr's notes of the post-colloquium meeting of workshop leaders, recorders, and Colloquium planners offer a critical assessment of the strengths and limitations of each of the sub-groups. The notes also included helpful suggestions for planning the next *Doris Siegel Memorial Colloquium*. Overall, the group's after-thoughts reaffirm the important function that the workshop component of the Colloquium format serves in meeting the purposes to which Doris Siegel dedicated her professional life and which the Memorial Fund in her name perpetuates.

Together, these documents represent the conversion of the oral history of the implications of change for members of the health and health-related professions, narrated by the workshops' participants, into the unabridged compendium of the workshop proceedings, written by the "think" piece authors and workshop recorders. Inevitably, some of the substance and style of the interdisciplinary discourse that informed the workshop effort has been lost in the conversion process.

The influence of this loss on the reliability and objectivity of the final report is compounded by the fact that the author's own firsthand experiences and subjective reactions to the continuing changes that have occurred in the health care environment since her halcyon days as Doris Siegel's naive social work student are inevitably reflected in her interpretation of the source materials.

In an attempt to do justice to both the process and outcome of the workshop deliberations and the relationship of one to the other, the report is divided into three separate but inter-related sections:

Section 1—describes and discusses the influence of continuity and change on the workshop agenda: the past-present-future connection as expressed in such important determinants of the process and outcome of interdisciplinary discourse as: (1) the workshop purpose, (2) the organizing principles that govern the arrangements for making optimum use of the four hours allocated to the workshop component of the Colloquium design, and (3) that most important determinant of outcome, the characteristics of the workshop population.

Section 2—describes and discusses the participants' response to the workshop charge as gleaned from the reporters' notes, the summaries of the "think" pieces that opened each session, and the post-workshop meeting. It identifies the common and different ways that the participants interpreted the cognitive and affective demands of the changing conditions of the health care environment, their respective strategies for coping with change, and their recommendations for addressing the future. A description of the effects of the interdisciplinary process itself on converting differences in interests, perspectives, and responsibilities into recommendations for affirmative interdisciplinary action concludes this section of the report.

Section 3—discusses the implications of the workshop findings for the on-going search for ways to reach the social-health benefits of modern medical care. The report concludes with the author's own assessment of the task that lies ahead as it affects the present and future "dispersal of power" among and between the health care professions and disciplines and the larger society.

HARMONIZING THE EFFORT

Modern society requires specialists, a differentiation of interest and objectives and therefore fails without pluralism. But it also needs to harmonize the efforts . . . so civil society needs constant organizing. (Lewis, 1990)

Section 1: The Work Agenda
in Developmental Perspective:
Linking the Past with the Present and Future

Both continuity and change are reflected in the workshop agenda. A re-reading of Dr. Rehr's introduction to the written proceedings of the first Doris Siegel Memorial Colloquium, *Medicine and Social Work: An Exploration in Interprofessionalism* (Rehr, 1974) serves to establish the linkage between the purpose, planning, and implementation of the 1988 workshop and the efforts of the Memorial Committee, charged with "formulating and planning the first project of the Doris Siegel Memorial Fund, to establish a level of professional excellence consonant with the vision of the Fund, to encourage and support social work in its efforts to enhance the social effectiveness of health and medical care." Invited by the committee to participate in the planning process by offering their suggestions for the objectives and format of the first Doris Siegel Memorial event, the "large numbers of social-health professionals who had contributed to the fund" strongly recommended a conference or colloquium dealing with the development of interprofessional social-health delivery systems both in practice and education.

The 1988 workshop deliberations thus continue the exploration of social work's relationship to the other health professions and disciplines in enhancing the social-health effectiveness of health and medical care that was set in motion by the first Doris Siegel Memorial Colloquium in April, 1973 in response to the expressed need of a large group of the social-health professional community of those times. The ensuing years and the changing conditions affecting the relationship of health and medical care to society have, if anything, reinforced the need for continuing this exploration.

The passage of time and its positive and negative influence on the conditions of the internal and external social-health climate not only affirm the necessity of continuing to "harmonize the efforts" of the various health professions and disciplines whose differences in knowledge and skills are essential to the identification and solution of social-health problems and/or issues. Time and the changing context of health care have also made it necessary—and more and more possible—to broaden the scope of the harmonizing efforts beyond the focus of the 1973 workshop agenda: the exploration of ways to overcome the barriers in health care practice and professional education that limited the effectiveness of social work's collaboration with medicine in the delivery of personal health services.

The latter-day workshop agenda thus takes into account the growing complexity of the social-health problems and issues now confronting the health and health-related professions, disciplines, and institutions; the growth and change in the knowledge, skills, as well as financial resources required for their identification and solution; and the concomitant necessity to encourage and support social work's relationship with colleagues from a growing number of health and health-related professions and disciplines in the broader range of activities through which contemporary health programs and institutions define and express their social-health commitment.

In addition to the consideration of the operational meaning of the changing context of health care for the present and future delivery of personal health services and the education of future members of the health professions, participants were charged with the responsibility for in-depth discussion of change and its implications for their present and future engagement in the following additional social-health related institutional responsibilities: the organization and management of social-health resources, the formulation of health policy, health planning, and regulation, and research and evaluation. Implicit in this broader charge was the need to explore whether and how their specific functional responsibilities affected the ways in which members of the *same* as well as *different* health and health-related professions and disciplines were likely to experience, react to, and/or interpret the effects of the changing context of health care on their exercise of social-health responsibility. Intra- and interpersonal and cross-functional relationships were thus implicated in this exploration.

Continuity and Change:
The Characteristics of the Workshop Population

Generational as well as professional and disciplinary differences were represented in the workshop population. Several attendees were veterans of the social-health action of the 1960s. The greater number, however, had embarked on their chosen health care careers in the aftermath of the changes in the relationship between medicine to society associated with the so-called "social-health revolution" of the preceding decade. They thus represented the post-1960s generation: a new group of health and health-related professions and disciplines whose professional growth and development had been shaped by continued exposure to the scientific, technological, social-political, economic, and demographic changes identified by the plenary speakers.

Regardless of professional, disciplinary, or generational differences, however, the workshop participants, like the participants in the earlier workshops, were selected on the basis of their ability to meet the following membership requirements:

- Their potential or already demonstrated capacities to speak for their respective profession or discipline, as judged by their mentors and peers.
- The high quality of their contributions to the advancement of the knowledge and resolution of health care problems and issues, as exemplified by their contributions to the professional literature and in the exercise of their practice, educational, and/or research responsibilities.
- The relevance of the knowledge, skills, and values of their particular profession and/or discipline to the overall purpose of the Colloquium and to the specific objectives of the small group sessions.
- Their special knowledge and experience in dealing with a particular subject area or health care issue encompassed in the workshop agenda.

Assessed in terms of the preceding characteristics, there is little to differentiate the general attributes of the latter day workshop participants from those of their predecessors. Continuity is thus expressed in the interdisciplinary nature of the population mix and the preservation of the same high standards of thought and action that have been represented in the workshop membership since 1973, the starting date of the Doris Siegel Memorial Colloquia.

Changing times and circumstances, however, were reflected in the differences between the size and geographic distribution of the 1973 and 1988 populations. The first workshop population was comprised of a nation-wide group of over 150 health care experts. Fifteen years later, growing constraints on the amount of release time and reimbursement of travel formerly provided by the participants' parent institutions made it necessary to confine workshop attendance to 60 health care leaders, drawn with few exceptions, from the east coast health care establishment. As a result, the character of the workshop changed from that of a large national conference to that of a much smaller regional meeting.

Despite this sharp decline in the size of the total population, social workers, as before, out-numbered the other professions and disciplines represented in the population mix. Size also made no discernible difference in the ratio of social workers to the non-social workers in either the workshop as a whole or the five small groups into which it was divided. A disconcerting number of "no shows" among those physicians who had accepted invitations to participate however, accounted for a regrettable and unexplained loss in what, in earlier workshops, had constituted a highly visible and vocal physician presence. Given the smaller size of the total population, it is important to note an increase in the number of social scientists among the non-social work representatives. By contrast, both the numerical and proportional representation of nurses declined. Health care consumers, as earlier, continued to be significantly under-represented.

The passing years appear to have had little effect on the institutional affiliations of the participants. In 1988, as in 1973, workshop attendees represented the professional staffs of medical centers and faculties of schools of medicine, social work, nursing, and graduate programs in the social, behavioral, and managerial sciences. Physicians were the most likely to hold both hospital and medical school appointments.

The effects of change on the characteristics of the workshop participants are most vividly illustrated by an examination of the nature and scope of their daily institutional activities—the experiential frame of reference that informed their responses to the workshop charge. Seen from this perspective, the 15 years following the initiation of the Doris Siegel Colloquia in 1973 have been characterized by continuous growth in the knowledge base of the respective health care professions and disciplines represented in the workshop membership, the development of new areas of expertise for addressing both new and persistent health care problems and issues, and new intra- and inter-professional alliances.

A review of the published proceedings of the first colloquium, for instance, indicates that most of the participants in the 1973 workshop deliberations represented the dominant mode of hospital based social work practice in the early 1970s: the planning, organization, and delivery of social-health services to the sick patients on the floors or in the specialty clinics of the nation's medical centers that represented their primary institutional affiliations. Only two were formally engaged in the planning, policy-making, and/or managerial activities of the particular institutions that they represented. Several were engaged in field instruction for graduate social work students; with the exception of the representatives of the Mount Sinai School of Medicine, responsibility for the education of medical students and residents was incorporated within the participants' delivery of clinical social work services. Involvement in research was minimal.

The social work educators among the workshop attendees were likewise engaged primarily in classroom teaching in the clinical methods courses of the master's curriculum and/or the human growth and development sequences. A few faculty members were responsible for the development of special concentrations in health care in response to the growing demand for social workers prepared to address the complex psycho-social problems of both hospitalized and ambulatory patients. Physician participants, for the most part, represented the prevailing model of the United States physician, circa 1973: the clinical specialist who combined hospital-based patient care and teaching with private fee-for-service practice. A smaller cadre of physicians represented the "new men and women of medicine," spawned by the short-lived social-health revolution of the preceding decade. A few of this group were engaged in the provision of primary care services in free-standing community-based health centers; a few others, in prepaid group practice. The larger number of this minority group were members of family practice or community medicine faculties. Their activities encompassed the planning, organization and delivery of primary health care services; health services research; and the epidemiological investigation of health problems in population groups.

By 1988, the social work members of the workshop population represented a broader range and different distribution of functional responsibilities. In addition to reaffirming social work's continuing engagement in the organization and delivery of hospital-based social services, the social work membership also reflected: (1) the

proportionate growth in the number of social workers now participating in or carrying major responsibility for institutional planning,
policy-making, and management; (2) the growing investment of social work practitioners in the systematic study of social work practice and the social-health needs of the various individuals and populations served; (3) the growing priority given to research
capabilities in the appointment and promotion of social work faculty; and (4) the growing involvement of social work in interdisciplinary collaboration in education, practice, research, and the formulation and implementation of social-health policy. Assessed in
terms of their career choices and their specific responsibilities, the
majority of the physicians who actually participated in the 1988
workshop closely resembled the members of the 1973 minority.
Many of the physician attendees combined administrative, teaching, and/or research responsibilities with engagement in clinical
practice. The fact that primary care practitioners, ambulatory care
directors, and physicians invested in health policy and health service research outnumbered tertiary care specialties may however be
due to the high "no show" rate among the physician invitees rather
than to a change in the behavioral characteristics of today's prevailing physician model. Neither valid inferences, nor, for that matter,
comfort can therefore be derived from this particular finding.

The composition and responsibilities of the membership of the
social, behavioral and managerial science component of the population reflected the growing number of the health-related disciplines
who combine academic responsibilities in graduate programs for
members of their own discipline with active engagement in the
planning, policy-making, research, and teaching activities of academic medical centers. While medical sociology was the only social science discipline represented in the 1973 workshop, the 1988
population also included the disciplines of health economics, an-
thropology, political science, and health care management.

The composition of the non-social work component of the 1988
workshop also recognized the increasing importance of the role that
epidemiologists are now playing in the general education of medical
students and residents and in interdisciplinary studies of the social-
health needs and problems of special population groups. The two
epidemiologists included in the workshop population were both in-

volved in promoting the linkage between population based medicine — the traditional province of public health and community medicine — and the care of the individual patient and family — the traditional province of clinical medicine.

With the exception of the limited representation of the responsibilities of nursing and specialty medicine, the major activities of the health and health-related professions and disciplines in the 1980s are reflected in the experiential frame of reference that informed the workshop deliberations. The small size of the workshop membership, coupled with the difficulty of correcting for personal, professional, and regional biases, limit the ability of the workshop participants to speak for the effects of the changing context of health care on the daily activities of the universe of health and health-related providers. Nor can the interpretation of the impact of change on the health care consumer expressed by the health care providers and the one health care consumer included in the workshop population — no matter how thoughtful and empathic — speak *for* or *to* change as it is experienced and dealt with in the real life of the universe of health care consumers.

The Workshop Arrangements

The workshop arrangements represent the results of the planning committee's efforts to create a modus operandi for facilitating in-depth exploration of the effects of change on the participants' exercise of their present and future social-health responsibilities. The workshop was therefore divided into five concurrent sessions, each focused on one of the specific functions encompassed in the overall workshop agenda and in the criteria for the selection of the workshop members.

To approximate the "real life" interdisciplinary mix in each of the five discussion groups, consideration was given to the participant's profession or discipline as well as his/her institutional role and function(s) in determining his/her particular group assignment.

The following sub-themes constituted the frame of reference for establishing the relationship between the plenary and workshop sessions and the relationship of the group sessions, one to the other:

— Reconciling past, present, and future.

— The changing demography and nature of health care problems.

— The impact of auspices on health care programs and reimbursement and financing patterns.

— Reconciling cost effectiveness with optimum social-health outcomes.

— Collaborative relationships.

The workshop plan designated co-leaders, a social worker, and a member of another health profession for each of the five discussion groups. Unforeseen circumstances, however, prevented three of the leaders from attending the workshop. Social workers alone therefore carried responsibility for the leadership of three of the discussion groups. The remaining two were co-chaired by a social worker and physician, in one case, and a social worker and health care administrator in the other. Social workers served as recorders in all five sessions. Because of the importance ascribed by the planning committee to the ability of both leaders and recorders to participate in establishing general guidelines for the conduct of the sessions in advance of the workshop, their selection was limited to the leadership of the health care educational and practice community of greater New York.

Selected on the basis of their established record as leading exponents of the social-health objectives of their respective institutional or program responsibilities, the authors of the "think" piece written in advance of the workshop, served as opening speakers and ongoing participants in the particular discussion group to which each was assigned. Their contribution to the process and outcome of the workshop will be considered in the second section of this report.

In concluding this description of the workshop agenda and the modus operandi for its implementation, it is important to reiterate that the committee's own thoughts, feelings, and experiences in dealing with change as a persistent demand of their membership in the health care professional community are deeply implicated in the overall workshop design.

Section 2: The Workshop Deliberation: Cross Functional Perspectives

The Workshop Climate

The workshop deliberations took place within sight and sound of the demolition, renovation, and expansion of Mount Sinai's physical facilities to meet the present and anticipated space requirements of scientific and technological growth and development and rapidly changing diagnostic and treatment modalities for addressing the complex health problems of the Medical Center's culturally and economically diverse patient population. The confusion and dislocation associated with building for the future provided a singularly appropriate backdrop for the consideration of the operational meaning of change to members of the health and health-related professions and disciplines.

The welcoming remarks of the workshop leaders, followed by the introductory statements of the "think" piece authors helped to create internal order in the midst of the chaotic conditions of the external environment. It was apparent from the spirited discussion set in motion by this "formal" component of each of the sessions that the participants welcomed the opportunity to exchange the thoughts and feelings generated by their personal exposure to change, uncertainty, and inconsistency as they were expressed in the conditions of their particular institutional environments.

Except for the workshop leaders and introductory speakers, no specific advance preparation was stipulated in Dr. Rosenberg's invitation to the other workshop participants. Nor were they given either choice or advance notification of their particular small group assignment. In selecting them for workshop membership, however, the planning committee had expressed their confidence in the participants' ability to draw on their rich store of knowledge and daily experience in service as expert witnesses to the implications of the changing context of health care for the present and future exercise of social-health responsibility. The planning committee was not disappointed. As the transcript of their testimony shows, the participants' response to the workshop charge, if anything, exceeded the committee's high expectations, bringing new insights to bear on the understanding of the effects of change on health system, provider, and consumer behavior and opening up new areas for continuing exploration.

Regardless of profession, discipline, or functional orientation, the participants' testimony demonstrated common concerns about the effects of change on their capacities to anticipate as well as respond to the changing health needs and expectations of consumers. Their self-assessment was characterized by a singular lack of defensiveness and an absence of narcissism.

The introductory statements and the continuing small group discussion addressed the particular themes identified as their charge in the workshop agenda. Their testimony indicates, however, that both the introductory speakers and the participants in each of the groups found the function-specific focus of their assignments too narrow for the full expression of the facts and feelings that informed their exploration of their particular charge. Much of their contribution to the knowledge and understanding of the circular relationship between external and internal forces in influencing the present and future social-health reach of their interventions thus evolved from the violations of the pre-determined boundaries of their assignments. In an attempt to convey the style and substance of their deliberations, the author's organization, description, and interpretation of the workshop proceedings also transgresses the functional boundaries, which as a member of the planning committee she had helped to establish.

Moving Backward on the Way to the Future: The Effects of Change on Institutional Behavior

Thus far in the collective experience of the participants in living with change as it was expressed in the life style of the particular academic medical centers or general hospitals with which the greater number of workshop members were directly associated, dollar-driven social and regulatory changes had served to reinforce rather than correct for the growing discrepancy between the institutional deployment of human and material health resources and the changing demography and nature of health problems and issues.

Like the physical facilities of their parent hospitals whose services were strongly implicated in government's cost control and containment initiatives, the ideological frame of reference that informed hospital spending habits, in the participants' judgement, also required renovation and expansion to promote and implement the integration of psycho-social with biomedical knowledge and technological inventiveness in addressing persistent, new, and emerging health needs and priorities.

In the course of the workshop deliberations, all groups considered the impact of institutional change for the exercise of their particular functional responsibilities. The main body of the evidence that attested to the symbiotic relationship between external and internal forces in shaping institutional behavior, however, was derived from the deliberations of those groups that explored the institutional functions most frequently cited in the bill of indictment charging the country's hospitals with fiscal mismanagement and social negligence:

— the delivery of clinical personal health services;
— the organization and management of social-health services;
— health policy, planning, and regulations.

Although the deliberations of each of the preceding groups led to the same general conclusions, the differences in the conceptual base, cognitive style, and experiential frame of reference of the health professions and disciplines represented in each group's membership were reflected in their perceptions of the specific ways in which the interplay between external and internal forces was expressed in institutional policies, programs and services.

Both the introductory speakers and participants in the session concerned with the delivery of clinical personal health services derived their perceptions of the effects of change on institutional behavior from their daily encounters with patients and families on the floors and clinics of their parent hospitals or in the privacy of their offices. Viewed from inside the hospital system, the heaviest burden of cost-driven changes in institutional policies and practices was carried by those members of the patient population least physically, emotionally, and/or socially able to carry it: the elderly, the poor of all ages, the chronically and terminally ill, the functionally incapacitated, and the growing number of patients hospitalized for the treatment of medicalized social problems such as alcoholism, drug abuse, child neglect, physical and sexual abuse, and more recently AIDS. For this group of high cost medical care utilizers, the concept of an "episode of illness" used to determine the reimbursement of the cost of a hospital stay for recipients of Medicare and Medicaid benefits was an oxymoron. Illness for them was likely to defy DRG specifications for a reimbursable length of hospital stay for a variety of social as well as biomedical reasons. For a growing number of patients and families then, the issue was not that institutional behavior was changing but that it was changing in the wrong direction. Aided and abetted by social policy and regulatory directives, the gap between their health care needs and the personal clinical health services provided by the hospital was widening, not narrowing. Access to and utilization of in-patient services was becoming increasingly restricted. As in the pre-Medicare/Medicaid days, the elderly and the poor of all ages were once again finding themselves more and more dependent on either their own dwindling financial resources or the hospital's dwindling charitable dollar to meet the costs of the overstay of their DRG welcome, even when beset by medical complications.

For far too many patients, the participants reported, the difficulties imposed by the limited social-health reach of institutional services were compounded by the changing conditions of the larger social environment. In the present, as in the past, the hospital has relied on the family and community to provide or supplement the post-hospital care for patients unable to meet their social-health needs without emotional support and/or physical assistance. At an earlier and, in retrospect an easier time, families were more able to serve their traditional function as the primary health care providers for the sick and functionally incapacitated. By the mid 1980s, however, both patients and families were perceived to require more help from home health agencies and long-term care facilities than there were equipped to give them.

Social work participants indicated that after-care planning for the majority of the patients on their "most difficult to discharge" roster had already been complicated by one or more of the changing characteristics of the American family described by Dr. Carol Meyer, a social work educator and expert in clinical social work theory and practice, in her introductory remarks that opened the clinically-focussed workshop session.

Many of the elderly and chronically ill or disabled patients awaiting hospital discharge were likely to be widowed women, living alone either by choice or by virtue of such personal circumstances as childlessness, geographic distance from their children's homes, crowded family living conditions, or, in many cases, a prior history of parent-child estrangement. A few of the patients, it was noted, had no home to which to return. At the point of admission, either they or their children had assumed that they would never be able to leave the hospital. Those patients living with children (mostly daughters) were dependent on care from members of the post-1960s generation of American women. These women were either working full-time or part-time outside their homes, sometimes out of necessity, sometimes out of choice. The majority combined their work life with the life of the traditional American housewife: child rearing, shopping, cooking, and cleaning. The older the patient the more likely his/her children were to be confronting the social-health problems inherent in their own aging process.

The case vignettes of children and adolescents needing post-hospital services provided, if anything, a more disturbing picture of family life for the chronically ill or functionally disabled child or teenagers living mainly in the medically and socially underserved neighborhoods of the inner city. The majority of the members of this growing population group were returning to either single-parent households mostly headed by mothers, or households with unrelated members — a roommate of the same or opposite sex, live-ins, and casual drop-ins. Their parent or parents were more likely than not to be teenagers, themselves often the victims of social deprivation, estrangement from their own families, alcohol and/or drug abuse, sexual exploitation, and increasingly AIDS.

Social workers attested that, for both the young and the old, current reimbursement policies had brought to the surface the long-time social deficiencies in the psycho-social services offered by the community as well as by the hospital. Indeed, in their judgement, "through the medicalization of social ills hospitals are being held responsible to assume a greater share of the burden, pushing responsibility beyond capacity to perform adequately.''

Based on the assessment of the status of community services, funding policies at the local, state, and federal levels offered few if any incentives for enhancing neighborhood-based primary care for the two most vulnerable populations in the life cycle, the young and the old. Public attitudes toward social-health problems associated with social deviance such as drug abuse, alcohol abuse, and AIDS have further deterred the development of neighborhood-based special programs for the prevention and treatment of these respective bio-psycho-social problems. Home health services, like primary care, were restricted by the disease focus of reimbursement policies. Long-term care for both populations was deemed inadequate for the needs of children as well as for the elderly. The collaboration between social agencies and health settings, which in their judgement was required for effective service to patients and families or to ''mobilize social action'', had deteriorated and indeed, had sometimes become adversarial. They agreed that true change in the current institutional model of care could only be achieved through a national health care system.

Strong affirmation for this conclusion and validation of many of the clinical observations on which it was based came from the opening speakers, a health economist, a health policy expert, and an epidemiologist and the physicians and social workers who constituted the membership of the workshop session focused on health policy, planning, and regulation. Their assessment of the factors affecting institutional behavior was grounded in economic, organizational, and population theory, the findings from their own research, and direct experience in institutional policy-making and planning as faculty members, consultants, and social work administrators in leading academic medical centers. Although distanced, for the most part, from direct contact with patients and families, they shared their clinical colleagues' deep concern for the effects of the current social and institutional climate on patients and families at high risk for medicalized social problems. As their testimony unfolded, the contribution of statistical compassion to the exercise of clinical compassion became more and more evident.

In their opening remarks to the participants in the social policy

focused session, both Dr. Charlotte Muller and Dr. Herbert Lukashok attributed the growing power of social policy and regulatory
changes to influence how health care institutions define and address
their responsibilities to the populations served, to the growing de-
pendency of the country's network of academic centers and general
hospitals on Medicare and Medicaid dollars for maintenance of
their fiscal viability. Hospitals in the 1980s thus have found themselves "faced with the inevitability of accountability to and oversight by third party payers and tensions between providers and payers."

Originally intended to do away with financial barriers of access
to health services for the aging and the poor, Medicare and Medicaid, through a series of modifications in their formula for the reimbursement of health services, appear to have lost sight of the need to
adapt their incentives to the changing health services required by
the elderly and the poor in order to remain true to their original
purpose. Instead, Medicare throughout its developmental history
has "continued to create incentives for activist rather than cognitive
care." The prospective payment formula for the reimbursement of
hospital services to Medicare and Medicaid recipients thus was
viewed as a continuation of this tradition. Its deficiencies in meeting the health needs of its beneficiaries were reflected in the findings of local and regional studies, cited by the introductory speakers, that showed that by failing to award post-hospital services and
primary care, the responsibilities and costs of after care had shifted
to families and community-based health and health related services.
Participants agreed that the architects of the latest incentives structure could not be held solely responsible for the limitations of the
medical model for the organization and delivery of health services
to the aged and the poor of today and tomorrow. At the same time,
however, they associated the tenacity of the hold of the medical
model on institutional behavior with Medicare and Medicaid's failure to provide incentives for loosening it.

While cautioning against the tendency to discount the tremen-
dous advances in treatment stimulated by the rewarding of "high
technology," Dr. Muller identified some recent trends that point to
the cost implications of seeming social policy and institutional com-
plicity in lowering fiscal costs at the price of disregarding the medi-

cal and social consequences of unattended social concomitants of illness and its care.

Anecdotal evidence and the findings of recent studies of the effects of institutional compliance with dollar-driven regulatory initiatives on the costs of hospital care, cited by the introductory speakers and the participants, suggested that the dollar savings accrued by shortening the length of hospital stay might in fact be an artifact of such reputed hospital practices as: (1) restricting hospital admission of patients (both the poor and the elderly) at high risk for protracted, and costly hospital stays; (2) transferring patients needing prolonged care from voluntary to public hospitals; and as previously indicated (3) shifting the costs of poor hospital care to patients, families, and community-based home care services and long-term institutional facilities.

The question of whether or not voluntary hospitals were guilty of "dumping" applicants for hospital admission whose medical needs presaged a lengthy hospital stay stimulated a lively debate among the panelists and the participants but no definitive resolution. The existing evidence tended to show that such differences as auspices, bed availability, and regional health care resources were likely to determine whether or not hospitals resorted to "dumping" practices.

The issue of rationing—considered by some participants to be a euphemism for "dumping"—also evoked a great deal of panelists' interaction. Although no official rationing policy had as yet been adopted, the participants agreed that "rationing by price" was already occurring, encouraged by the PPS incentive to "treat less, not more." The implications of this practice for the aged and the poor as the population who have been consistently identified by epidemiological studies as being at highest risk for prolonged and costly hospital stays was a matter of deep concern for all participants.

Rationing by age, it was pointed out, had already been proposed by leading public figures in politics and bioethics as a solution for dealing with the growing evidence that the biggest cost of care is associated with the end of life. The ethical conflicts inherent in this proposal, which has received a great deal of professional and popular media attention stimulated on-going discussions focused on the following areas, cited verbatim from the reporter's minutes:

— "The use of resources/investments to prolong the lives of those with little productive futures as opposed to the use of these resources for other medical and social programs for which economic and social productivity would be the result."
— "Ethical conflicts about treatment choices of decisions to prolong life in the face of biomedical technological advances for those who have survived into old, old age. These decisions have often pitted the elderly and their families against the medical care system."

The following forces were identified as contributing to the medical care system's encouragement of the prolongation of life even in the face of a deviating public: medical training; the defensive practice of medicine; a reimbursement system in New York State which rewards nursing homes with higher rates for the more dependent and debilitated and for prolonging lives; a social-cultural uneasiness about the discussion of death and dying, preventing the elderly from making their wishes known.

In this, as in other value-laden issues affecting the rationing of services on the basis of age, it was generally agreed that:

1. functional capacities rather than chronological age should be the determinant of the treatment choices offered to the patient;
2. patients or their named surrogates should be given the final choice of determining the nature, extent and duration of life-sustaining medical interventions.

Although perhaps most dramatically expressed in the discussion of institutional policies and practices with respect to death and dying, the conflict between consumers' health needs and preferences and the criteria for determining for what purposes and for whom the health care dollar was spent emerged as the major source of the participants' dissatisfaction with present social policy and regulatory directions.

The participants agreed that what they perceived as needed change in health policies and practices to correct for DRG-created barriers to access to care and for limitations in the scope and quality of institutional services could not be accomplished through tinkering with reimbursement strategies without dealing with the "medical/social needs" that they exacerbated.

They thus recognized that changes in health policies alone would be insufficient to deal with the crisis they identified as confronting the health care system in the present and not too distant future. Public policy deficiencies in dealing with such prevalent social problems as poverty, broken homes, family strife, and increasing homelessness had already been converted into increasing demands for the medical treatment of social problems among high-cost health care utilizers. Nonetheless, they joined with their clinical colleagues in their general endorsement of a national health insurance system as a first step in correcting for the social-health deficiencies of the existing public and voluntary medical and social services and programs.

The author has purposely left for last the description of the meaning of changing social policy and regulations for the "doers" of new and changing policy and regulatory directives: the health care professionals who carry the responsibilities of reconciling the social-health needs of the aggregate population(s) served by the hospital with the needs of the individual patient in the organization and management of social-health resources. In contrast to the participants in the social policy focused session, the introductory speakers and participants based their perceptions of the institutional response to policy and regulatory change on their own direct involvement in coping with change as their assigned responsibilities rather than on "institutional and organization theories and/or empirical studies."

The four introductory speakers of this workshop were: the director of a social service department in an academic medical center; the physician in charge of ambulatory pediatric services in a large inner city teaching hospital; a social work faculty member and expert in substance abuse; and a consultant in health care management. The participants represented social workers and physicians, who like their counterparts in the speakers' panel, carried managerial responsibilities as part of their designated departmental or program responsibilities.

The general tone of the introductory statements and the discussion they evoked, as gleaned by the author from the "think" pieces, reporter's minutes, and Dr. Rehr's summary of the post-conference meeting with the workshop leaders and recorders, was more accepting of or perhaps more resigned to the conditions of the institutional environment and less social-action oriented than that of the previously described testimony of the clinically and policy-focussed sessions. While the participants addressed many of the same issues as their colleagues in the two other sessions, their major emphasis was on the identification of ways to bring about change within the system through the innovative use of existing institutional and community health and health-related resources.

To the director of the hospital social service department of an academic medical center, the increasing emphasis of the hospital administration on cost effectiveness and efficiency presented an opportunity to accomplish her long time objective: to change the organizational structure for the delivery of social services from "four independent sections of social work for OB/GYN and Perinatal Medicine, Medical/Surgical, Psychiatry, and Pediatrics" to a centralized social service department. Ms. Breslin's introductory remarks provide a vivid example of the effects of organizational change on not only social work but institutional behavior.

The process of "recreating social work's departmental identity" coincided with the introduction of the prospective payment system in her hospital. As a result, the department's present activities have been shaped by an "evolving series of changes in the health care industry, which provided the opportunity for social work to participate in the implementation of our hospital's business initiatives that have continued to reflect us as a caring medical setting and a collaborative community health resource."

The importance of networking with a growing number of community groups was also the major theme of the introductory statement of the director of ambulatory pediatrics services. Dr. Grimm's remarks focused on the importance of interdepartmental collaboration both in addressing child health needs and problems and in maintaining staff morale in dealing with serious social-health problems as they present in the population served by an inner city medical center. The interdisciplinary activities that she described again call attention to the range of problems that fall outside the services covered by Medicaid benefits to the poor and their children. She cited the following examples of interdisciplinary efforts to address

neglected areas of social-health needs that were represented in the
pediatric population served by the hospital and the community:

- — an interdisciplinary committee to monitor operations of the
  emergency rooms;
- — child protection meetings which on a weekly basis deliberate
  over cases of suspected child abuse and neglect;
- — a city-wide child protection committee which looks at broader
  issues of child protection and in essence becomes a negotiating
  committee with such governmental agencies as Special Services for Children;
- — a special care clinic for children with AIDS, children of sub-
  stance-abusing parents and parents with psychiatric problems,
  and children who are victims of child abuse or neglect;
- — a pediatric chest clinic which provides comprehensive care for
  chronic lung disease and asthma;
- — a school outreach program which joins pediatricians, a nurse,
  and a social worker with educators and school administrators
  in the development and implementation of school health services.

The third member of the speakers' panel, a social work educator
with special knowledge and expertise in the planning of services for
the prevention and treatment of alcoholism, called particular attention to the ethical and economic implications of the growing investment of hospital resources in the treatment of persons with medicalized social problems. Like the participants in both the clinically
and policy-focused groups, Dr. Saunders noted that hospitals were
being asked to compensate for society's lack of responsiveness to
those who engage in "self-destructive" behaviors. Health care professionals, in his experience, felt powerless in dealing with what he
termed "socially-negative disease." Using alcoholism as an example of a prevalent problem that is viewed by the public and many
members of the health professions as created by patients' deviant
behavior, he described a proposed model for a state wide consor-
tium that would join the resources of the state's colleges and univer-
sities in a unified program for "training and dissemination of information on alcohol and other drug problems" in order to broaden

public understanding of problems of substance abuse and enhance the quality of programs of the treatment and rehabilitation of the growing population of substance abusers.

As the final introductory speaker, the hospital care consultant placed the efforts of program and department managers to make optimum use of health and community resources in the larger context of the current struggles of the hospital to reconcile the multiple demands that compete for attention with the cost control and containment imperative. In common with the members of the social policy-oriented group, Ms. McGoldrick acknowledged the powerful role of auspices and incentives as determinants of institutional decision-making. Dollars, she reiterated, play a critical part in today's service delivery. The reach and quality of services are therefore driven by the funding agency. She concluded with her belief that the current trend to shift costs from public auspices to business, and increasingly from business onto consumers would not be deterred without changing the fee-for-service system.

The discussion that followed, like three of the four introductory statements, was micro-patient focused rather than organizationally related. Although no unifying theme was identified or pursued, the deliberations convey a sense of the commonly held social values of the participants, their commitment to patient centered social-health services, and a capacity to find creative ways of joining health care resources with those of the community in the interests of equity and economy.

While different in scope, substance, and functional frame of reference, the three sessions that addressed the implication of change for institutional behavior as a major component of their deliberations complement rather than contradict one another. As a cross-functional assessment of the social-health strengths and limitations of institutional behavior under social and economic stress, their conjoint testimony provides important insights regarding the multiple factors that affect the institutional capacity to respond to change in ways consonant with the goals and values inherent in a social-health definition of institutional responsibility. Overall, their assessment highlights the importance of understanding the dynamics of institutional behavior as a prerequisite for interdisciplinary efforts to broaden the scope and enhance the social effectiveness of institutional programs and services.

Reversing the Direction of Change: The Participants' Examination of Their Own Behavior

Functional orientation, as previously noted, made a considerable difference in the amount of time and attention devoted by each of the groups to the exploration of the relationship between external and internal forces in shaping institutional behavior. Not so with respect to the participants' allocation of time and thought to the explanation of the implications of change for their own behavior, their relationships with one another and with members of the larger community: health care consumers and providers of health and health-related home-based and institutional services. It was clear from their deliberations that the opportunity to discuss their own responses to change and ways of enhancing the social effectiveness of their interventions was a principle reason for their investment of uncompensated time in workshop attendance.

In the process of their self-examination, each group addressed the following questions at some point in the course of their inquiries:

— What are the cognitive and affective demands of external and internal change on the daily exercise of their assigned institutional responsibilities?

— What are the areas of consonance and dissonance between the ideology of social, political, and economic change and the standards of excellence and accountability inherent in their respective behavioral codes? ·

— What are the strengths and limitations of their own capacities (knowledge, skills, and attitudes) to respond to demographic and social policy and regulatory changes in ways consonant with their social-health values and aspirations?

— How ready, able, and willing are members of the health and health-related professions and disciplines to take the risks of loss in autonomy and territoriality inherent in the collective exercise of social responsibility?

— What changes are required in the prevailing model of health and medical care that will promote and enhance the optimum

use of human and material health resources in expanding the scope and enhancing the social effectiveness of health and medical care interactions?
— What changes will be required in interdisciplinary behavior in , order to optimize the contributions of the health and health-related professions to a generic social-health model for expanding the social reach of health and medical care?

The reporters' minutes and "think" pieces suggest that, of all participants, members of the clinically focused session expressed the strongest affective reactions to the demands of cost-driven changes in institutional rules and regulations on their own behavior and the satisfaction derived from the daily practice. The introductory remarks of Dr. Mack Lipkin, a primary care physician and medical educator, speak to the feelings expressed by the group in the discussion that followed his presentation:

> A number of factors are increasing tensions within each of our disciplines. To some extent this is a health-system-wide problem. As this occurs, the ability of a discipline to see beyond its borders decreases, tribalism increases, territoriality heightens.
> The principal driving force for this is the perception, and it is the perception that is the key, not the reality (which is bad enough) of diminishing resources. As people are anxious concerning their share, they are less generous in sharing.
> There is in the health professions a feeling of heightened loss of control. It is a kind of helplessness and it can be pervasive. It derives in part from the nature of the work which faces helplessness every day in tragic situations. But it also comes from the outside. Bureaucratization is rampant. The average primary care physician spends 20% to 25% of effort in doing paper work.
> Recently there seems to be less to go around of status, money, responsibility and authority, and tender loving care. When one feels that one's status is diminishing it is a hard time to be asked to share it with those who would like more.

Participants in all sessions, including the clinically oriented group agreed that what was perceived as a growing sense of dissatisfaction with the outcomes of their efforts to affect as well as respond to change was exacerbated by the deficits in their knowledge and skills in addressing the cognitive demand of change. As was true of the group's perceptions of the effects of change on institutional behavior, the membership's perceptions of the cognitive demands of change, although derived from a functional frame of reference, also tended to complement rather than contradict one another.

Clinicians acknowledged that the mandate to make optimum use of health resources in the interest of cost efficiency had reinforced the importance of their capacities to: (1) identify patients at high risk for long hospital stays at the point of admission; (2) provide services to families as well as patients in planning for the post-hospital care of those patients needing continuing help in the management of their health problems; (3) establish linkages with community-based home care and institutional services to supplement or substitute for the patients' and families' care-giving functions.

Demographic changes and the changing nature of the problems of high cost health care utilizers also make a demand on their ability to make a distinction between the needs of the patients with acute versus chronic health problems, the health needs of the aging, and the old-old versus the child and the teenager. Changes in bio-medical knowledge and technology made a steady demand on their understanding of the effects of new and emerging treatment modalities and outcomes on patients' and families' planning for the post-hospital continuation of care. These changes also make particular demands on the treatment teams' ability to help patients and families understand and adapt to the medical and social sequelae of such dramatic therapeutic advances as open-heart surgery, organ transplant, and chemotherapy. Finally, rising cost-consciousness had awakened the clinicians' interest in prevention and health maintenance as modalities for reducing both the fiscal and social costs of illness. This interest was experienced as an increasing demand for understanding of the principle of epidemiology and health economics on which to justify the investment of clinical resources in preventive and health maintenance interventions. Participants in the session charged with exploring the implications of the changing conditions of the institutional environment for the organization and management of social-health resources experienced the demands of change as tests of their capacity to stretch the social-health reach of the health care dollar through: (1) adding business perspectives to traditional strategies for the allocation of deployment of finite human and material health care resources; (2) including social work positions in the "cost of doing business" when certificates of need were submitted to regulatory agencies; (3) collaborating with community services in the provision of case finding, outreach, and case management services; (4) establishing linkages with business and industry in providing a resource for meeting the growing need for employment assistance programs; (5) developing similar contractual arrangements with municipal governments.

Thus far, the description of the ways that participants perceived the cognitive demands of change in the exercise of social-health responsibilities has focused on the experiential evidence on which the two groups most directly associated with the organization, management, and delivery of medical care services based their testimony. Social workers and physicians in these groups indicated that they relied heavily on on-the-job learning to compensate for what they identified as deficiencies in their professional preparation for meeting the demands of new and changing policy and regulatory directives, new constraints on spending habits, and new and emerging changes in the health problems and demographic characteristics of the patients seeking their services.

The two sessions that explored the behavioral demands of social policy, regulatory, and planning functions and research and evaluation respectively, while sharing their practice-oriented colleagues' concerns with the effects of external and internal forces on the social-health outcomes of health and medical services, placed the behavioral demands inherent in addressing these concerns within the conceptual frames of reference that informed the dual responsibilities of: (1) interpreting the social-health and social cost implications of policy, planning, regulatory, and demographic changes; and (2) expanding and correcting for the limitations of the knowledge base on which both the interpretation and evaluation of social-health costs and outcomes and the factors that influence the scope and social effectiveness of health and medical care interventions are based. A fine thin line distinguishes these two functional responsibilities from one another. In both their real life experiences and in their workshop deliberations, the participants frequently crossed it. Their perceptions of demands were thus influenced by hands-on experience in research, teaching, and consultation as well as theory.

Seen from the perspective of the health economist, political scientist, epidemiologist, social worker, and physician who constituted the population mix of these two separate but inter-related sessions, clinical judgement, often based on intuition, reason, authority, tradition, sometimes mythology, and "too often dogma," Berkman thought they lacked the conceptual power and methodological rigor required "to inform principles of practice or generate action."

Although by intent, the major focus of the research group's deliberations was on ways to enhance the quality and scope of social work research, there was growing recognition that, for such important purposes as informing social action and movement of political processes, the development of operational measurements for the study of social costs, collaboration with health economists, political scientists, and epidemiologists would strengthen and add new conceptual dimensions and authority to the work.

A special need to encourage medical and social work practitioners and students to become informed research consumers as well as investigators was identified not only by the social policy and research-oriented groups but recommended as an essential requirement for addressing the future by members of the clinically-oriented session.

Dr. Hans Falck, a leader in social work research and education spoke to the need as a generic requirement for all members of the health professions in his opening remarks to the research group:

> We are now at the point in the various professions where research is considered fundamental to the improvement of their knowledge base and practice. Unfortunately, medicine has performed brilliantly but has produced far too few practitioners in the world-at-large who have learned enough research methodology to guide their daily practice. But that is also the case of the practicing social worker, nurse, and others. In

other words, while each profession has its superior producers of research, we are not yet at the point where practitioners are routinely able to integrate them into on-going practice. The ability to do this demands skills and knowledge of an advanced order and cannot be routinely produced by the kind and quality of continuing education offerings characteristic of other professions.

In the discussion that followed his opening statement, participants emphasized that the development of a "research attitude" was essential to the capacity "to integrate research knowledge into work with patients." "In an era of accountability," they indicated, "the task of practitioners becomes the same as the researchers, i.e., to give a logical account of what they have done. That means that practitioners should document failures as well as successes." In this, as in the preceding sessions, honesty and the ability to acknowledge one's biases were identified as essential requirements of professionalism.

Four groups demonstrated these attributes in the assessment of their capacities to deal with the demands of change in terms consonant with the values of their respective professions and disciplines. More attention was given to attitudes and values than to intellectual capacities in their assessment. As implied in Dr. Lipkin's previously quoted remarks, the demands of change for interdisciplinary collaboration brought to the surface unresolved issues of physician dominance among social workers and nurses. These were particularly evident in the discussion of the delivery of personal clinical services. In this, as in the other sessions, physicians and social workers also confronted the gap between their avowed belief in the involvement of consumers in decisions affecting the nature and extent of treatment interventions and their actual decision-making behavior. As Dr. Saunders' opening remarks to the session on the organization and management of social-health resources had pointed out, social workers and physicians alike admitted to their difficulties in dealing objectively with patients with self-destructive medical problems. Both the clinical session and the session devoted to the social policy, regulations, and planning also brought out biases toward or against other population groups among clinicians and policy-makers. These biases were particularly evident in discussion of the needs of children versus the needs of the aging and the aged. While intellectually participants agreed that age should not be the criteria for either the allocation of health care resources or the investment of professional diligence, competence, and social-health concern, their discussions of both rationing and other ways of dealing with the rising costs of person care indicated that like the general public and its elected officials, some workshop members thought that the growing costs of care for the aged would deprive the young of needed health care services in the present and the near and distant future. Others were equally concerned about what one participant termed "elder bashing."

What emerged with particular intensity and repetition were overt expressions of tensions, disagreements and perceived status differentials among members of the same professions. Physicians committed to prevention and primary care decried the dominance of specialists in health affairs and were particularly sensitive to the issue of incentives as it affected both the reimbursement of patient care and their own services. (The previously noted absence of representatives of the clinical specialties in the workshop population robbed them of the opportunity to speak in their own defense.) Reminders of the needs and benefits to be derived from bio-medical knowledge and technological inventiveness came, interestingly enough from social scientists and social workers. Here the need to distinguish between overuse and the appropriate use of biomedical and technological awareness was emphasized.

By far the most frequent feelings of estrangement, elitism, and disappointment were articulated by representatives of the clinical community — physicians and social workers — toward members of their respective educational and research communities.

They faulted the research and educational establishments, however, for different reasons: the former for ignoring their contributions; the latter, for failing to anticipate and/or meet their needs. Of the charges against the respective establishments, those leveled against education were more frequent and more specifically stated. Physicians represented in the groups emphasized the limitations of the bio-medical model of medical education in preparing them for understanding either the social context of health and medical care or for developing the skills required for the assessment of the social and psychological needs of their patients as essential factors in the diagnosis, treatment, and outcomes of their interventions. Social workers most frequently referred to the discrepancies between the academic curriculum and the learning demands of real-life practice. Like physicians, they felt that the broader social context of health care had been insufficiently addressed in their professional education to provide a conceptual frame of reference for understanding the relationship of health care services to the particular populations and communities they served. While more confident than physicians in their capacities to assess and deal with the social and psychological needs of individual patients and families, they felt far less adequately prepared for the conceptual and methodological demands of converting their assessments of the adverse social-health effects of policy and regulatory changes on the individual patients and family into empirical evidence on which to recommend and influence changes in institutional and governmental policy and regulatory initiatives.

Nor did they feel sufficiently grounded in the principles and methods for assessing and dealing with health problems in population groups to inform the activities associated with proactive social work behavior: consumer education; collaborating in the design and implementation of programs for the prevention, early detection, and treatment of medical and medicalized health problems; the development of partnerships with community-based health and social agencies, business, and industry in the provision of health maintenance and preventive services.

How did the particular medical and social work educators who comprised the membership of the group charged with the responsibility to address the implications of change for education of the health professions assess the needs of their students and their responsibilities to meet them? Had the participants in the other group been able to eavesdrop on the educationally-focused session they would have heard academicians voice many of the same perceptions of the demands of change for a new generation of medical and social work students as they had defined on the basis of their experience. With few exceptions, however, representatives of the academic community tended to place more emphasis on broadening the knowledge and skills required for enhancing the psycho-social effectiveness of clinical practice than on strengthening the capacities of practitioners to influence institutional social policies and regulations, participate in institutional decision-making and the administration of patient care services, and/or develop the knowledge and skills on which to base preventive interventions.

These differences in their emphasis from that of social work and medical practitioners in the other groups is implicit in the final statement in the reporter's minutes, summarizing the areas in which the educational group reached consensus:

> Health care policy has had through regulation and will continue to have an enormous impact on how care is organized, delivered and also on patient/professional autonomy in terms of decision-making. Given this, it is important to also ensure that all professions have some understanding of policy and its implications for practice.

On the other hand, however, the educationally focused deliberations were more exclusively devoted to the exploration of the interdisciplinary demands of present and future education for medical and social work practice than any of the other sessions. While all other groups discussed the issue of interdisciplinary behavior as a major theme of their respective function-specific assignments, medical and social work educators represented in the educationally-focused group devoted most of the allocated time for the workshop component of the Colloquium to revisiting one of the central themes of the workshop sessions included in the first Doris Siegel Memorial Colloquium — the exploration of interprofessional education for future physicians and social workers. Like their academic colleagues of an earlier day, their discussions placed the demands of educating for the exercise of the interdisciplinary responsibilities of medical and social work practice in the context of the larger educational, institutional, and social environment. In common with Dr. Lipkin, whose opening remarks to the participants in the clinically-focused session emphasized the need for an "interactive science informed by a psycho-social approach and a generative spirit of caring," the academicians too, recognized that "psycho-social knowledge belongs to everyone." "It is in the doing," they agreed, "that knowledge becomes unique and specialized to a profession" or within specialty and sub-specialty groups.

In making the distinctions between core knowledge and common knowledge, the group pointed out the rapidity with which core knowledge was changing. What was once unique to the knowledge base of a profession has become part of their common knowledge pool and more and more a part of the public knowledge domain. What the group considered important for each profession to know, understand, and accept in one another were each other's particular claims to the common knowledge base and the differences in the ways each applied his/her knowledge to an interdisciplinary mode of thought and professional action. The group also concurred that no profession had an exclusive claim to the attributes that expressed the "generative spirit of caring." The art of listening to patients and families in decisions affecting the conditions, extent, and duration of medical treatment; the maintenance of high standards of care through processing new and changing biomedical as well as psycho-social knowledge were therefore identified as the common demands for learning and teaching the behavioral requirements of an interdisciplinary model of social-health caring.

In the process of exploring issues of commonality and differences among health professionals, with particular reference to the way medical and social work education prepared their students for a changing social-health future, social work members of the group reached the disconcerting conclusions that medical education has been quicker to acknowledge, albeit still ambivalently, the role of psycho-social factors in the cause, course, and outcome of disease than social work education to make space for biological concepts and principles in the conceptual frame of references for assessing and dealing with medical and social problems.

As the result of this exchange between social work and medical educators, questions began to emerge with respect to the ways "we are taught or not taught to assess each other's expertise." In addressing their questions, participants made a distinction between "taught" and "caught" learning. In their crucial position as role models for future physicians and social workers, they were sensitive to the fact that they represented an important component of the "caught" learning derived from the hidden curriculum on which much of student learning about values and attitudes toward patients, families, and colleagues from other professions and disciplines is frequently based.

As the environment of health care had become increasingly stressful, subject to outside controls over university as well as hospital spending habits, participants acknowledged that the task of controlling their own feelings of competition with colleagues for a fair share of curriculum time, research funds, and/or academic status was becoming more and more difficult. The maintenance of student morale and belief in the value of their own chosen profession as an essential component in the socializing process inherent in the educational function was also seriously threatened by daily confrontation with the limitations of medicine and social work in altering the adverse medical and social consequences of medicalized social-health problems rooted in poverty, homelessness, racism, and parental and societal indifference and/or neglect. Students were also increasingly exposed to the faculty's struggles to deal with the bioethical issues that have followed in the wake of the dramatic achievements of biomedical science and technology. All in all, these were not positive times for serving as role models of objectivity and certainty.

In his opening remarks to the education-oriented session, Dr. Howard Zucker, a medical educator holding a joint appointment on the faculties of medicine and psychiatry, summarized the threats that change posed for the realization of the personal hopes and expectations of both the health care consumer and provider and the ways that they evaluate and value each other's behavior in the following statement:

> Maintenance of morale is central in preparing for change. In the larger world economic and ecological limitations and pressures will, during the next 30 years or more, be expressed in social unrest, governmental upheavals, and rebellious outbursts by those who in reality have unmet basic health needs

and who in fantasy believe that new governments or new heroes will rapidly make complex problems disappear.

In the smaller world of the health care professions the same tendencies are active. We are likely to experience powerlessness, depression, and fury as we are forced to accept changes in our life style, self concepts and professional identities. It is easier to blame other people and groups for these painful changes than to adapt to large impersonal forces — and by scapegoating to increase feelings of alienation. I see a lot of depression, anger, and demoralization in the health profession today.

Like Dr. Zucker, the other participants looked to the development of continuing dialogue among the health professions as the way to help ease the problems and initiate "useful innovations that will bring back some of the satisfaction and fun to our work which so many now find to be missing." Strong support was therefore given to faculty development as an essential component in opening up opportunities for broadening the scope and effectiveness of interdisciplinary collaboration.

As the participants began to share their own ideas and experiences in dealing with change, the workshop itself began to take on the characteristics of a faculty training and development session. Concerns about how each of the professions valued each other seemed, at least temporarily, to have been laid aside as medical and social work educators began to grapple with persistent issues that, as Dr. Carlton, a social work educator indicated in his opening remarks, had confronted social work education throughout its developmental history — the relationship of education to practice.

Medical educators pointed out that this issue was not unique to social work education. Indeed, it is deeply embedded in the recommendations for curriculum reform recently issued by the Association of American Medical Colleges. Dr. David Cohen, a health care administrator with particular knowledge and experience in graduate education in primary care, pointed out that efforts to make medical education more relevant to practice had also characterized recommended reforms and new accreditation standards for residency training.

In discussing the specific ways to strengthen the capacity of health care practitioners to address the changing health needs of the patients and families they served, they acknowledged the need to "educate clinicians and researchers as well as individuals who can integrate the knowledge into the conceptual whole." They also agreed that "any model of interdisciplinary practice needs to include the patient/family/community as part of the work group. The issue of longitudinal/continuity of care was discussed and recognized as essential. In order to address this last issue, both individual as well as system interventions will be recognized."

Although the concept of integrating the faculty within the academic environment with the faculty within the practice environment was raised as a possible approach to reducing dissonance between academia and the field, no specific recommendations for bringing such an integration about were made. Nor was specific consideration given to identifying those disciplines other than social workers, physicians, and to a lesser degree nurses, needed to design and implement an interdisciplinary model for medical and social work education that would broaden the social-health reach and effectiveness of interdisciplinary interventions.

The following themes were discussed in the group's exploration: (1) problems in interdisciplinary practice, (2) content for interdisciplinary education, (3) the academic-practice relationship, and (4) model of interdisciplinary education. The reporter's minutes identify areas of consensus reached by the end of the spirited interaction between the introductory speakers: a social work educator, a medical educator with a particular investment in humanistic medical education and practice, and a medical educator and health care administrator with a particular interest and experience in graduate medical education for primary care practice. This imbalance between the representation of medical and social work education on the introductory speakers' panel was compensated by the skills of the leaders, a social worker, and a medical educator in involving the recorder, a social work member of a medical school faculty, and the other participants, mostly social workers, in what under their leadership became a round table discussion.

To the participants, the optimum expression of interprofessionalism in interdisciplinary practice was adversely affected by "conflicting and contradicting messages in the health care environment between staff, between staff and patients, and between the staff's and the institution's interpretation of organizational goals." Health care providers, in their judgement, often do not have common definitions of what team work, collaboration, or consultation are. The "myths" that surround interdisciplinary practice "often interfere or prevent it from happening." The group suggested that perhaps the concept of working groups rather than teams more accurately reflected the "diversity of roles and responsibilities and thus contributions of each professional to health care."

Unresolved issues from the past with respect to "who coordinates patient care, namely acts as the leader of the work group or team" were raised in the familiar discussion of appropriate ways to assign team leadership to non-physician health professionals arose in the course of the discussion of the role of the patient/family in the interdisciplinary process. Questions were raised as to whether the patient/family could be helped, or even allowed a leadership role. The "ideal" arrangement, identified by the participants, was a partnership between patient and health providers. Parenthetically, it should be noted that the implications of the partnership model for educational providers and educational consumers were not discussed in the on-going discussion of ways to relate education to the participants' perceptions of an ideal model for clinical practice.

Educators agreed that as health providers, physicians and social workers have not done a good job with tools they have such as decision analysis, epidemiology, etc. in terms of educating the patients about choices for care nor "have professionals been educated to use these tools."

Self awareness of the factors of one's own behavior that promote or interfere with one's behavior as a member of an interdisciplinary group were discussed in the context of the prevailing conditions of the health care environment. There is little difference between the following statement, excerpted from the reporter's minutes of the session and Dr. Lipkin's statement to the members of the clinically-focused session, quoted earlier in this report: "Many felt that increasing regulations, the issue of malpractice, were making professionals self-conscious to the point that there was demoralization among caregivers as were a sense of immobilization and often overtreatment of patients."

In considering the "content" to be included in a model of interdisciplinary education for the delivery of patient care, the participants focused on such critical educational questions as: What is unique to what social work, nursing, and medicine do? How are these differences expressed in educational autonomy (the issue of turf) and in the socialization process for members of the respective health professions?

In ending this descriptive analysis of the deliberations of the educationally-focused session, the author calls particular attention to the similarities and discrepancies between the preceding group's perceptions of their educational needs and aspirations as these emerged in their discussions of the social-health mandate of the present and the future and the perceptions of needed changes in basic and continuing social work and medical education expressed by the members of the academic communities of medicine and social work, represented in the session devoted specifically to the exploration of interdisciplinary education.

As indicated in the description of their interactions with one another, the introductory speakers and our other representatives of the academic community demonstrated a sensitivity to the affective demands of change on both faculty and student relationships with one another that, in both substance and intensity, mirrored the feelings expressed by social work and medical practitioners engaged in the daily delivery of care to patients and families. Educators, perhaps because of their own need to keep up with changing knowledge in their fields as a condition of imparting knowledge to others, were also empathetic with the intellectual and subjective demands of change and uncertainty, generated by the persistent need to process new and emerging concepts of health, disease, and human behavior in assessing patients' needs and in determining appropriate treatment interventions, while coping with the changing conditions of the health care environment.

Like their colleagues engaged in clinical practice, research, and social policy and planning, they too were deeply concerned with finding ways of enabling students to understand and address increasingly complex ethical problems and issues, particularly those decisions affecting the nature and extent of life-sustaining medical intervention.

Medical educators more than social work educators acknowledged the need to prepare the future practitioner for the responsibilities of primary care through the provision of residency and fellowship training opportunities. Neither social workers nor medical educators, however, gave more than peripheral attention to ways of addressing the need—expressed by participants in all other groups—to strengthen their capacities for developing and implementing proactive interdisciplinary strategies, including a stronger voice in social policy and system change. Nor did their identification of the key elements to be included in an interdisciplinary model of medical and social work education address the cognitive demands associated with the cost-effective organization and management of social-health resources, identified by both health care managers and social policy and planning experts in their respective sessions.

Perhaps, most important however, educators were deeply aware of the tension between education and practice and were committed to finding the ways of reducing it. Their deliberations pointed up sufficient areas of agreement on which to have further explanation of those areas which reflect differences in their perceptions of the demands of change for present and future social-health practice.

Section 3: Changing the Social-Health Context of Interdisciplinary Collaboration: Implications for Future Health Care Providers and Consumers

Although the workshop participants, with few exceptions, indicated their awareness of the power of adversity—as expressed in dollar driven health system behavior—to reawaken or evoke feelings of competition, loss of professional territoriality and/or control of their own destiny, there was little evidence of interdisciplinary disharmony in their workshop behavior. In fact, it was only by reading the roster of workshop attendees or references to their own profession or discipline in specific comments cited by the recorders that the author was able to distinguish the professional or discipli-nary identity of the participants in her review of the reporters' min-utes.

If a "sense of the common good," as Lewis suggests, is essential to harmonize the benefits of socialization, then the behavior of the workshop participants suggest that the threat of the changing con-text of health care to their capacities to act in the best interest of health consumers was a motivating factor in enabling the partici-pants to place the charge to their particular workshop sessions within an interdisciplinary frame of reference.

In contrast to the state of interprofessionalism as reflected in the relationship of social work to medicine described in the proceedings of the first Doris Siegel Memorial Colloquium, the physicians rep-resented in the 1988 workshop population associated the attributes of social workers with the distinguishing characteristics of the so-cial work profession rather than with the attributes of "their particu-lar social worker," the designation most commonly used by 1973 physician participants as the referential base for their assessment of social work behavior.

The blurring of territorial boundaries between medicine and so-cial work, described in the 1973 proceedings as a major cause of discussion between and among members of the traditional health care teams — doctors, nurses, and social workers — appeared to be accepted as a reality and indeed a source of potential strength by physicians and social workers represented in the 1988 workshop population. There was some indication, however, (although there were far too few nurses in the population mix to affirm or deny it) that nurses were increasingly involved in a struggle to establish their autonomy and rights of eminent domain in health and medical affairs.

What emerges with striking clarity is the participants' growing recognition of the needs and the rights of health care consumers to act in their own best interest, rather than relying on health care providers to act for them. Whether discussing the delivery of per-sonal health services, health policy, and regulating and planning issues, on the organization and management of social-health resources, the health care consumer was acknowledged as a neglected resource for the discovery of ways to enhance the social-health effectiveness of professional services. Educators, along with practitioners, indicated that an interdisciplinary model for education and practice should include the health care consumer as a member of the work force for interdisciplinary functions and responsibilities.

The 1988 workshop deliberations also indicated that practitioners among the workshop participants had overcome much of their earlier resistance to broadening the scope of interdisciplinary interventions to include a greater investment in the development and implementation of preventive, health maintenance, and case management services in collaboration with community-based health and health-related programs, services, and long-term care institutions. Educators, however, as previously indicated, had failed to recognize the cognitive and affective demands of proactive interdisciplinary behavior in their projected design of an educational model for interdisciplinary educators.

While more similarities than differences characterize the response of the participants, when viewed in terms of their functional rather than professional or disciplinary orientation, the fact that the differences suggest a continued dichotomy between education and practice, and a perceived status differential between knowledge builders and knowledge consumers, including members of the academic as well as practice community points to the need for on-going intra-disciplinary and functional exploration among members of the health and health-related professions and disciplines.

By recent action of the National Association of Social Workers' Board of Delegates, a recommended proposal for a national health insurance system was strongly endorsed by the professional association of United States social workers. Business and industry are increasingly recognizing that issues of economy and equity in health care coverage of the American worker cannot be achieved under the present fee-for-service system. There are gleams in the political eye that the inequities of access and limitations of services generated by the PPS reimbursement system have not gone unnoticed. The consumer's rights to know and to decide in matters affecting the circumstances of his/her living and dying have slowly but surely gained legislative and judicial credibility. There are encouraging signs that the social-health context of interdisciplinary collaboration is slowly changing, partly by a re-gathering of the external social forces that influence system behavior, partly because of the adverse effects of dollar-driven initiatives designed to control rising health care costs, and partly because of the courage and creativity of sung and unsung heroes and heroines in the first pages of the next chapter of health system development.

What remains as a cause for continuing concern, even in the deliberations of a highly selected population of leading health care thinkers and doers is the failure to close the gap between the demands of change as perceived by practitioners and educators.

In his opening remarks to the participants in the session devoted to health policy, planning, and regulations functions, Professor Lukashok pointed out that "final decisions concerning which investments to make depend in the long-run on the values the individual and society desire—these are human—not technical decisions."

To the author this is an appropriate note on which to conclude this description and analysis of the process and outcome of the workshop deliberations and to indulge in a few personal comments on the values for patients, families, and the health care system that can be derived from an on-going exploration of the factors that promote or interfere with the capacity of members of the health and health-related professions and disciplines to harmonize their differences in the interest of the collective exercise of social-health responsibility.

What emerges clearly in the joint testimony of the participants in the 1988 workshop is the need for the professions and disciplines to respect and value themselves as a prerequisite for respecting and valuing the knowledge, skills, and experiences of the growing number of significant others—consumers as well as health care providers—who make up the extended health care community. Self respect and self-value to the members of the extended health care community comes from a sense of competence as well as commitment; these beliefs in one's own worth and ability come as well from a recognition of one's usefulness by peers, professional and disciplinary colleagues, and consumers—students as well as patients and families. They are affirmed through institutional policies and practices that encourage and recognize involvement in decisions affecting the social-health environment of health and medical care, as well as the conditions of one's own professional life as a member of the institutional community.

Without the internal supports that come from the way that professional education exercises its responsibilities for socializing its students to the values and behavioral norms of their respective professions; the external supports that come from recognition of competence by colleagues and satisfied consumers; and demonstrated institutional trust in the professional's capacity for self-government, taking the risks involved in changing institutional, societal, or interdisciplinary behavior becomes problematic, and too often, not worth the taking in terms of social-health outcomes.

Interdisciplinary collaboration, if it is to be worth this arduous investment thus begins at home in the ways that members of the same profession or discipline are prepared and rewarded for respecting and valuing intradisciplinary collegiality.

REFERENCES

Flora Lewis "Needs of Civil Society," (Op Ed Page) *The New York Times,* August 8, 1990.

Helen Rehr (Editor) *Medicine and Social Work: An Exploration in Interprofessionalism,* Prodist, New York, 1974.

Part IV

*Conclusions
and
Recommendations*

Social-Health Care:
Problems and Predictions

Helen Rehr
Gary Rosenberg

INTRODUCTION

We have a health care crisis in the United States. We have an epidemic of social problems as well. If we are to seek solutions to both crises, a national integrated social-health policy is needed. Given the serious problems in our social-health and personal behavior systems — fragmented and limited access to health care, poverty, homelessness, hunger, AIDS, substance abuse, person abuse — we cite the urgency for national social-health planning and ask:

- How serious do our social problems have to become, before we make these the highest priority for action?
- The efficiency and effectiveness of the American health care system has been challenged. How do we make it effective and functional?
- Are the problems resolvable? What measures are necessary?
- Restrictive conservatism and immediate past and present policies have contributed to the problems. Will the policies continue or will we have a renaissance of humanitarian liberalism, building on the Roosevelt through the Johnson periods?

Whatever is done the resolution will affect "who gets what, when and how." The policies adopted will affect social programs,

Helen Rehr, DSW, is Professor of Community Medicine Emerita, Mount Sinai School of Medicine, City University of New York. Gary Rosenberg, PhD, is the Edith J. Baerwald Professor of Community Medicine (Social Work), Mount Sinai School of Medicine, City University of New York.

the health care system, and the means to implement and support them. Any changes will cost more than spending levels today, and much of the expenditures may need to be reallocated based on priority determination and strategy. Most public polls indicate that the majority of Americans are willing to support essential social services for the needy, and a universal health care system for all.

This chapter deals with some of our major social-health problems, the changing health and health care patterns, and offers some conclusions and recommendations relevant to health while noting the relatedness of health and social ailments.

BACKGROUND

The right to health as an American ideal has been passed over as illusory and unachievable in a world of social turmoil, inequities, and of dissimilarities in individuals, cultures, and nations. If the "right to health" is unachievable, then another American ideal is forthcoming, "the right to health care." The way to "health" in individuals requires more than political and public financial actions. An individual's life-style, socio-economic situation, genetic background, environmental exposure, and available health care are also major contributors to his/her state of health. If this premise is accepted then it is apparent that social and personal welfare and health are interrelated, and planning would require viewing these factors together. In this context the availability of dollars does affect what can be done in the public arena and those actions can affect the health status of people. Today, the right to basic health services does not exist for large numbers of Americans.

Until 15 years ago, social and public health history reflected a slow but steady incremental change in the welfare of the American people. Since World War I as a result of major public health measures, such as anti-malarial care, immunizations, antibacterial drugs, and water treatment, more people have enjoyed more positive health effects than from direct medical care (Thomas, 1977). There has been no political controversy over the fact that public social welfare measures such as child labor laws and health programs, which have required either passive or mandatory compliance (seat belts), have been the more effective "stay healthy" preventive measures.

In reviewing the 40-year history from the Great Depression to the 1970s, a wide variety of national social and health policies have been supported by moral and social obligations of Americans, which have had major effects on public well-being:

- Social Security in the mid-1930s has been a boon to the elderly, the unemployed, the disabled, children, and others in reducing poverty via its age-related and unemployment insurance components, and its grants for public health and for social services to the states;
- The Veteran's Administration health and social support programs after World War II, followed by Medicare and Medicaid and more child health programs in the 1960s — all federally implemented — assured access to veterans, the aged, the poor, and particularly children and their parents to health services, and aided the indigent elderly to meet nursing home needs. Over time these programs had expanded to add selected and other needy populations at-risk. They have been accredited with enhancing the general health status and even the life expectancy of Americans (Rehr and Rosenberg, 1986, p. 77-78);
- Supplemental Security Income (SSI) for the needy poor and Title XX are support programs to the states for comprehensive social service programs and further support to Social Security recipients via cost of living adjustments (COLA's) to deal with inflation (Estes, 1989).

However, the 1980s brought major changes in policy. Reagan conservatism was furthered by a fiscal crisis, and with it came a taxpayers' revolt, which resulted in capping outlays and frank cutbacks in support of existing social benefits. The major change in national health policy of the 1960s to that of the 1980s has been from one that pledged national commitment of all governmental efforts to assure high quality comprehensive health care, to a so-called "safety net" of limited services for the most deprived (Rehr and Rosenberg, 1986, p. 80).

Under the Reagan Administration, health care has been reshaped. A shift in policy in 1981 moved responsibility for the payment of services to the individual. The Reagan era pressed for increasing cost to the elderly for Medicare covered services by larger deductibles and increased premiums, for cutbacks in federal matching of state funds, for support of Medicaid, for primary care, and for maternal and child health services (Davis, 1986, pp. 40-43). While the evidence is still out on the long-term effects of the Reagan strategy in regard to social and welfare programs—there is evidence of health deterioration among selected at-risk populations (Davis, 1986, p. 43). The fact that more than 37 million Americans are without health insurance is sufficient to indicate the threat to the health and quality of life to a large number of our population—the poor, minorities, and the most vulnerable—the majority of whom are under 65 years of age. Additionally,

- another 25 million people are underinsured, in particular the blacks and Hispanics who lacked steady health care coverage over a 28 month period ending May, 1987 (AHA Washington Watch, April/May 1990, p. 12);
- over two-thirds of these uncovered or marginally covered persons are workers employed in small business or service organizations with no or inadequate health care benefits (they are the working poor);
- almost 12 million children under 18 years of age are uncovered for health needs—including one out of seven adolescents (Hospitals, August 20, 1989, pp. 14 and 25);
- those over 65 years of age—12% of our population—use 40% of hospital days and only 45% of their health care bill is paid by Medicare; 3% of Medicare beneficiaries use 46% of Medicare costs (Meyers and Masters, 1989, p. 200); Medicaid covers a considerable part of their medical costs, but a substantial component is paid out-of-pocket or by private insurance; medical care costs the covered elderly 8% of their household incomes (Davis, 1986, p. 39);
- 5% of the elderly are in nursing homes, the majority on Medicaid (Weiner et al., 1989, p. 91); many of the nursing homes

have been cited for questionable care, and corrective legislation is pending in Congress; "most disabled elderly are currently cared for at home by family without any paid services." (Weiner et al., 1989, p. 89);

— over 33 million people were hospitalized in 1987, an 11% decline over 5 years, but most are sicker—in particular, the elderly and the poor—in shorter lengths of stay than before DRG's, and with an inadequate number of community support services to assist with their post-discharge "at home" needs;

— while hospitalizations are down, outpatient visits are up and 75% are by those seeking help for their anxiety, fears, depression, and worries (Rehr, 1983, p. 256);

— the extent of poverty in the U.S. is a social and moral disgrace; homelessness is fast becoming an epidemic; and hunger is prevalent among the homeless and the unemployed (Reuler, 1989);

— substance abuse is rampant among all age groups, while each year more of our youth become affected;

— AIDS is the number one infectious disease—HIV positive cases are expected to grow to over 3 million in the early 1990s, killing thousands each year, unless a curative drug is found; the AIDS problem is no longer solely a homosexual problem, but heterosexual as well, and associated with drug abuse;

— our failing educational system does not produce a literate youth ready to fit into the needed labor force of today and tomorrow, nor knowledgeable enough to stay healthy;

— air and environmental pollution are out of control; waste disposal, including chemical and nuclear contaminants, is without resolution for all regions in the U.S.;

— an exploding aging population by the 2000s, at two extremes of health: many remaining well, while those who are ill will be sicker than today with greater disabilities;

— mental illnesses occurring in staggering numbers;

— chronic illnesses and their sequelae affecting 65% of the American public; the elderly are the most afflicted;

— accidents and injuries resulted in over 59 million acute conditions in 1988, or 24.6% per 100: 1 out of every 4 people in the

U.S.; and are the 5th leading cause of death (National Center for Health Statistics, 1988);
— violence and people abuse — children, women, and the elderly — have surfaced in such numbers as to be overwhelming.

Many of these social problems described are significantly American. There are more, which, when viewed collectively, reflect a public policy of piecemeal social and health programs that have in no way diminished the problems and the numbers of people who endure them. The relationship between the social welfare of our people and their health is clearly evidenced by the current social-health status of the American people.

HEALTH CARE AND HEALTH IN THE U.S.

In 1987 Americans paid $500 billion for health care. This amount is expected to rise to $600 billion in 1989, approximately 12% of the G.N.P., and constitutes the highest expenditure for health services of all westernized nations. We spend 100% more per capita than the Japanese and 50% more than the Canadians. Americans spend an average $2,000 per year for health care while the British spend $500 on average; and yet our mortality and morbidity rates are comparable to theirs (Lamm, 1989, p. 4). Also, over 50 million people under 65 years of age have inadequate insurance coverage or are without any protection at all (Glasser, 1986, p. 64).

There are those who raise concern whether the 12% of GNP, which goes to health costs, is efficiently used (Ruddick, 1989, pp. 161-163). Many economists cite waste and unnecessary procedures in health care delivery; even fraud and abuse have been uncovered among providers. Overuse and invalid consumption by large numbers of people are not uncommon as they translate stress, fear, and anxiety into medical visits, or are encouraged to excessive visits by over-zealous medical personnel.

The economic crisis of the 1970s and the soaring costs of all social programs as well as for medical care, came one on the other, created an explosive impact on budgets at the federal and state levels, and resulted in outcries to cut back sharply. Wage increases and new technology in the health care industry, together with more people becoming eligible for and using covered services, contributed to bursting the dollar bubble.

A first attempt to deal with the fiscal crisis was directed at hospitals. Cost controls were introduced by the federal government in 1972 through utilization review regulations, which attempted to regulate length of stay in the hospital. Industry, growing more and more concerned with the accelerating costs of health care for its employees, began to seek its own cost-cutting measures. In addition to introducing employee cost-sharing plans through deductibles and co-insurance, industry began to look for new ways to deal with health care delivery that would be less costly.

Most social and health care costs for the needy were thrown on the states. The states facing their own fiscal crisis followed with constraints imposed on services. Subsequently most third party payers imposed greater deductibles, higher premiums, or cutbacks in coverage.

The fiscal crisis hit the hospitals as early as the mid-1970s when they were expected to monitor utilization of services and to find ways to deal with runaway costs. The Professional Standards Review Organizations established under the 1972 Social Security amendments prescribed the monitoring and review of care delivered by providers—presumably a quality of care measure. However, its major function was to set up systems to "determine whether care has been provided at a level which is most economical" (Miller, 1983, p. 91). While there were denials of reimbursement under the new PSRO review mechanisms, the benefits hospitals and providers derived from the per diem and procedures reimbursement methodology slowed any gains from implementation of utilization review. However, in the mid-1980s when prospective payment was introduced for Medicare beneficiaries based on diagnostic related groups (DRG's) of diseases, changes did occur. Hospitals found that reimbursement for a "length of stay" was no longer based on in-hospital days, but was now diagnosis related, controlled by mandated cost containment of services. The new method of payment was meaningful in the reverse—a shorter than allowable stay would now be profitable while extended stays would be costly to the institution.

Medicare patterns of payments to hospitals under Part A, and to doctors and other covered services under Part B, and the new procedures, changed health care delivery. This Medicare type payment coverage to hospitals was adopted by most other third party payers.

Another major program impact on health care came as a result of deregulation, which also changed the health care system as we had known it from the Flexner period in 1917. A major commercialization of health care was added to the mix of voluntary teaching, community, and municipal and governmental hospitals. Hospitals had been the center of medical care supported by a range of fee-for-service professionals in the community who were generally attached to institutions. Deregulation fostered a burst of for-profit health industries that came into the marketplace as competitive enterprises, and added a third tier to the existing two tier system. The traditional two tier system — voluntary and municipal hospitals — was relatively equitable in whom they served. Both admitted Medicaid and Medicare recipients, the insured, and even a marginal income population with limited or no resources. The payment for care for those with little or no coverage traditionally had been underwritten by a long-term pattern of charity. In later years this shifted to a charitable cost factor, which was included in the reimbursement rates by the third party payers. However, with the commercialization or privatization of medical services, the traditional institutions faced a practice by the "for-profits," which tended to "cream" the private paying or "well-insured" patients. It was not unusual to find that the "creamed" patients were less sick than the medically indigent sick, frequently requiring shorter hospital stays, and as such were cost beneficial to the commercial institutions. At the same time the voluntary and municipal hospitals were impacted with costly services for the very sick. Hospitals were suffering from reduced income and began to find they had less and less resources to cover the non-paying group. The voluntaries, too, began looking for ways to seek out insured patients, and to transfer the non-payers to overburdened municipals.

As the fiscal crisis impinged on all levels of government, the states began to impose restrictions on medical care for the indigent.

Many put limits on the number of visits to out-patient services; many capped the number of hospital days that would be paid per year.

In setting limits, states were exercising a form of rationing of health care. Changes in benefits and services were made. As costs continued to rise due to price escalation and to the volume and intensity of care, the public evidenced some interest in some rationing of esoteric and of very expensive new technology, while it remained supportive of basic services for the needy (Hospitals, May 5, 1988, p. 79). As examples, both Oregon and Arizona, which had been covering the funding for bone marrow, pancreas, heart, and liver transplants, decided to legislate the reallocation of those limited monies to the support of prenatal care for low income mothers. As costs continued to rise, the governments (federal and state) imposed a rationing of care—witness the uninsured and the underinsured who have been without basic health services. It has been noted that people without health care coverage tend to face a medical crisis by delaying medical attention, and then by utilizing the emergency services of institutions, frequently in advanced states of illness (Glasser, 1986, p. 66) that tend to cost more than basic medical care.

The DRG's, utilization review, and the fiscal crisis brought the occupancy rates of hospitals into the political limelight. A major result was forcing the closing of beds (and hospitals) when occupancy rates remained low. An empty bed is a cost-factor since staff, supplies, and general maintenance have to be continued irrespective of the bed utilization. In New York State for example, where lower occupancy rates were occurring, the State forced the cutback of more than 5,000 beds. By the middle of the decade, as the AIDS crisis hit New York City hard, it faced a shortage of beds to serve those AIDS patients who are acutely ill, needing immediate care, and those terminally ill needing hospice and specialized services.

The DRG's have indeed contributed to reductions in the average length of stay. Since its introduction, there has also been a major shift to the utilization of ambulatory care. Even though there have been sharp reductions in hospital admissions and inpatient stays (20% decline since 1980), overall costs continue to rise for hospital care. There has been serious concern that the overconcentration on a prescribed "length of stay" has made a sicker in-hospital population more visible than before the DRG's because the earlier patient mix of sick and less sick has changed. Serious consequences have been reported when health care providers are expected to serve such a heavy concentration of seriously ill people with quality. In addition, there has been evidence that a number of patients may have been discharged prematurely—i.e., quicker and sicker—having to face the limited provisions in their communities for "at home" support services. Early discharge tends to shift the costs of post-hospital care to an outpatient status and to the patient and support network directly. While there may be hospital cost savings to payers what remains to be seen is the extent of savings from shortened inpatient stays. Shortened stays will need to be viewed alongside direct costs in the provision of formal services at home and in particular when the indirect social and financial costs to family members are added (Ancona-Berk and Chalmers, 1986). However, there is no question that being at home as early as possible is for most discharged patients a desirable outcome of the implementation of DRG's. While the intent of cutting the length of stay in hospitals was to force the closing of unneeded beds and hospitals, the growing AIDS epidemic has thwarted that intention. A shortage now exists where hospital beds (and hospitals) have been reduced in major and middle-sized urban areas.

As companies saw the costs of their health care benefit packages rise each year—greater than the Consumer Price Index—they have grown more concerned with its impact on the cost of their products and their competitive position in the marketplace. In 1988, Chrysler spent $700 on employee health care for each vehicle manufactured, twice as much as the French and the West German auto makers and three times as much as the Japanese (Califano, 1989). Businesses are responsible for about 25% of America's total health care bill; Federal, State and local governments for about 40% (in tax dollars); and individuals pay about 33% through insurance or direct payment. There have been new cost savings patterns introduced by the large companies in which they expect their employees to participate in the payment of health services for themselves and where applicable for their family members shifting from the 'everything' package to a consumer's limited choice from a menu of benefits. Deductibles and co-insurance payments are becoming commonplace.

There are other ways industry is attempting to cut or control its costs for health care. Many have introduced in-house direct or referral services though employee assistance programs as a means to control or direct what the employee gets in the way of care. Also managed care programs supported by industry, either in-house or purchased commercially, manage the care sick individuals receive. The care is often with pre-selected providers who are expected to save costs to the industry. A similar cost saving method is the PPO, the preferred provider organization, which contracts with industry for fixed price services, and employees are expected to use the PPO rather than selecting their own providers. The cost-saving health care benefits industry is currently proposing have become key issues in labor/management negotiations.

Hospitals, which have been the major source of health care because their services have been paid for by third party coverage, have been undergoing marked changes. The health care industry can no longer assume that there will be a market for inpatient services in the same way doctors had used hospitals for their patients before the changed reimbursement patterns. There is evidence that the traditional acute care patterns have changed. Hospitals must redefine their roles and functions in the health care enterprise. Most acute care hospitals now face that 50% of their inpatients are or will be over 65 years of age suffering from chronic illnesses (usually more than one) and thus frequently they must deal with both disease and age-related problems. The hospitals are becoming tertiary care centers with linkages to smaller community hospitals for referral and/or transfer of patients. Rehabilitation in both the physical and social functioning context is an early-initiated major component of inpatient services or for planned after-care.

In order to meet their financial needs hospitals are challenged to find new revenue producing enterprises and new systematic ways to deliver care. New technology, for example, in surgical procedures for cataracts and kidney stones has proved helpful in shifting inpatient care to one day ambulatory surgery. While there may be savings in hospital costs, the financial and social costs invested in suitable after-care supports to safeguard the surgical benefits have not been calculated in the overall costs of care (Ancona-Berk and Chalmers, 1986). Other approaches to cost savings have been the merger of two or more institutions. Sharing resources, curbing duplication, and avoiding overlapping services in a geographically connected area have proved helpful. Usually such joint ventures create a larger pool of prospective clientele for the arranged services of the institutions. The greater advantage in addition to cost savings to both institutions, is to the smaller one as it links to the larger, usually an academic setting, which makes available a range of services: clinical, management, educational, and research supports, that it did not have before. These nonprofit multi-hospital systems now control over one-quarter of the inpatient beds in the United States (Rehr and Miller, 1983, pp. 261-262).

As the non-profit institutions merged for survival and enhancement, they found themselves competing with a growing for-profit medical industry. The for-profits have not only entered the hospital care field but have moved steadily into a range of other health care programs. They have made a substantial commercial penetration into long term care programs, e.g., Marriott has opened retirement health care centers, claiming it is an expert in hotel services and can buy the health care components. They have entered the medical supply, the "at home" service, alcohol abstinence, mental health, and a host of other services for the aged sick and the disabled homebound.

Data indicate that one-fifth of those over 65 require a period of home care with a range of services at some point in time each year. For that 5% of the frail elderly who require institutionalized care, $35 billion was expended—50% by individuals and families, 43% by Medicaid, and a small percentage by insurance. There appears to be a trend in which patients who can afford it are responding by shifting to private care centers, paying for them by either insured or direct dollars, because they say they experience a more personalized service. There are critics of these new operations who have raised questions about the quality of medical care in commercialized enterprises (Relman, 1980). However, the voluntary hospitals have attempted to catch up and move ahead by entering into similar health enterprises and even non-health related ones such as hotels, spas, and restaurants. The hospitals have seen the need to broaden their concept of health care from the inpatient focus for the sick to anything that has to do with health maintenance. The hospital is becoming a multi-service health center drawing on its multiple expertise. Specialty centers are being developed, such as a Women's and/or Children's Social-Health Services Center, which encompass everything from medical intervention, social services with a range of counseling, to health education and maintenance programs. Such centers would and do include human services programs ranging from health promotion to becoming active participants in local and regional public health actions alongside the consumers of their services. They are also helping their consumers to become involved in community council type enterprises where key issues — not limited to health concerns — that are socially and politically relevant to the community are discussed and acted upon. There is a growing commitment to retrain health care providers to involve their patients (and the lay community) in decision-making about their care by creating a partnership between provider and consumer. Consumers are also participating in decisions for newly projected services in a given institution. The personalization and the individualization of care attributed to the for-profits are basic values subscribed to by more and more providers.

Linking or networking among community social agencies is becoming very important since joint programs can add supportive and educational services for the sick, their families, and in the promotion of health maintenance. Medical institutions have developed a range of health education programs, which they take into their local communities with the support of local residents. Hospitals have come to understand that they must be available for the elderly, young families, children, and the newborn for their present and future needs. "More than three-fourths of all Americans born in the last decade can expect to reach 65, even assuming no further improvement in mortality rates" (Longman, 1989, p. 135). Not so incidental is the staggering impact on Social Security for covered services for those who are insured. The longer life expectancy, which we are already enjoying, raises particular concern regarding whether it will be with quality. Quality lifestyles will be most critical both in terms of what the very young are exposed to now and when they reach old age. Marc Lalonde (1975, pp. 29-30) has noted that there are four areas that affect an individual's health status. They are human biology, the environment, his/her lifestyle, and the health care system. The hospital as a health care center is or will be interested in all four aspects. Currently some of the health education programs affecting lifestyle are in anti-smoking, anti-drug and alcohol, enhanced nutrition programs, education in regard to sexually transmitted diseases directed at both the adult and school age populations.

Medical care institutions, voluntary or commercial, are changing. Their missions have shifted to cover social-health care needs by diversification and through new organizational approaches. The shift is to place the major emphasis on a prospective client population — individual, groups, and their own employees — by reaching out to the social, educational, and industrial arenas with recognition that the target is not only the individual but his/her family as well (Melum, 1989, pp. 67-72).

While the new emphasis is on the young and the well our changing social demographics require a new view of how professionals deliver health care and how they perceive their clientele. More women are in the work force than ever before — 51% of them are mothers with children at home. There are more elderly entering their eighth decade. How do we keep the children, tomorrow's adults, healthy, and keep the 80-year-olds and older in as good health as possible? The cost for adequate prenatal care for a pregnant mother to deliver a well baby is an average $400 versus $1,000 per day for intensive 8-18 days of care for a low birth weight baby (Hospitals, July 5, 1989, pp. 52-54).

In addition to focusing on the young and the well and their health maintenance, the health care enterprise will of course continue to be concerned with those populations at-risk for serious health problems. Western societies must deal with chronic illnesses and their sequelae, and what is an epidemic of social diseases, ailments, and disorders.

Chronic illness is a significant factor in American society, despite scientific efforts to uncover their causes. Diseases of the heart, the circulatory system, cancer, the neurological and muscular debilities, and diabetes are still treated in an acute, palliative, and rehabilitative context, while the chronic disease itself continues as a constant recurring threat to the individual. The severely retarded and the developmentally disabled make up another substantial at-risk population to which one adds those suffering from chronic emotional distress or fatigue. Compounding these physical and emotional chronic ailments are a growing range of social diseases, which derive from self-styled destructive behaviors. Excesses in smoking, alcohol, drugs, and eating, along with accident-prone or promiscuous sexual behavior contribute to the social ailment group. One of the critical concerns we are currently facing derives from sexually-transmitted disease or from drug abuse practices. AIDS and HIV-infected individuals and infected newborns are fast be-coming the most overwhelming medical and social problems we face today. Unless a cure is found, AIDS and HIV infections will be the number one epidemic in the next decade—taking billions of dollars to meet treatment and service needs. There is more violence and uncontrolled drives in "too many" individuals resulting in per-son abuse of the elderly, women and children. How do we deal with these and other behavioral alterations in people? We must affect the educational system from the entry point and reinforce content throughout, while re-educating the family as well.

RECOMMENDATIONS

In Bess Dana's synthesis of the workshops' deliberations, the participants have reinforced the O'Leary and Friedman presenta-tions in identifying the many social and health problems Americans face in a turbulent society with finite resources. O'Leary empha-sizes the need to achieve quality in a rapidly changing health care environment. Friedman urges equitable access to care for all; sees changing professional and paraprofessional roles, particularly for women and minorities as the health care system undergoes a change from its male, white dominance. Both speakers are concerned with professionals' willingness to self-examine or peer review their prac-tice. They see a need for a systematic way to achieve case (patient care) assessment, and to secure good data and information so as to affect our policies. Both believe that educated consumers, and a trusting and true partnership of consumers and providers could make a major difference in the nature of direct services, and in broad policy deliberations.

Both O'Leary and Friedman were optimistic about the future. All involved in the Colloquium believed they see us coming out of a decade in which the government and the public have been deaf to the needs of the disenfranchised, the underclass, and the poor. The public is moving from an ultra-conservative me-ism of the 1980s to a more open and caring position. People want their representatives to find a more positive agenda than we have had, one that is more responsive to the needy. There is growing recognition that the past decade of deregulation, loosely defined competition and commercialization of social utilities, social and health supports, shifting costs to individuals and to state and local governments, has contributed to the chaos in our society. Small government cannot do the job alone and individuals are prepared to contribute a fair share for fair and just policies. A sense of outrage is growing in the middle class, which will be critical in voicing the need for change, the need to be more socially-oriented, to have concern for self and others in the future, and in the quality of health care services available to us.

POLICY, PROGRAM, EDUCATION, AND RESEARCH

Have excessive and rising costs of health care and the need to curb them played havoc with our ability to plan and reach sound public policy? Has an overconcentration on our outlay to institutions and to providers overlooked the public and their basic, essential social-health care? Have the deregulation and the commercialization of health services benefitted the public? Does society have a social and moral obligation to support the tenet "the right to health care" for all our people? Should hospitals be for private consumption in deregulated competition or are they a social utility to serve the public in its needs?

In general, health policy in this country has been medically-focused on institutions and doctors. It is our belief that our future requires a social-health policy that is based on people-related needs. As Friedman notes there is no unilinear relationship between cause and effect when illness strikes. There are many factors at work. It becomes more of a mosaic of problems (causes) that need to be addressed at many levels before finding positive outcomes.

The public welfare will be addressed soundly when the social welfare and health care are seen for their effect on each other. It may be somewhat strange for health care professionals to place their primary emphasis on the need to deal with poverty. The poor suffer more of all illnesses, have less access to health care than others, come into care later, are homeless and hungry, and suffer higher morbidity and mortality than other groups. The underclass derives from poverty and suffers more social ailments. Poverty and ethnic minorities have a high correlation. The first item on our national policy agenda has to be the elimination of poverty. There are a host of social problems such as substance abuse, mental stress, and air and environmental pollution, all of which correlate positively with available health care. Access to health care, basic and essential, for millions needs to be made available. Access is one of the most critical social issues. Hospitals have not been able to keep up the volume of uncompensated care as reimbursement sources were cut. Many have imposed barriers to entry and to services. Philanthropy, while available, cannot meet the costs of the growing demand on institutions. Access is associated with poverty, but more with the marginally poor who are without insurance or a public health care coverage, and with the working poor who are underinsured. By and large, the Medicaid program does cover most of the basic needs of the very poor although caps and limits on services have been imposed by the states as the federal government cut back its support of Medicaid. For all Americans, a national health insurance coverage is socially and morally correct. We are moving in that direction albeit piecemeal and with faltering first steps. The public has been supportive of care to those who are without resources.

AHA's President, Carol McCarthy, says change is underway. It would be foolish to overlook the continuing escalation in American health care costs in spite of reduced hospital stays and a shift to ambulatory care. There is something wrong with a system that does not cover 12-15% of Americans. McCarthy notes the number of national health insurance or health plans under discussion. Massachusetts has introduced a worksite coverage plan whereby employers would insure their employees with state support for small businesses and for coverage of basic services to the unemployed. This is a universal coverage for state residents (Hospitals, Aug. 20, 1989, p. 25).

Congress is grappling with a business support system for all employees and a broader base Medicaid program. There were a number of plans before Congress in 1989 dealing with basic health benefits for all Americans (S. 768). The bill would require employers to provide health insurance coverage for all their employees and their dependents. The uninsured and special business support for employers with limited employees would be provided for via a state business risk pool. Economists and health planners are looking to the Canadian National Health System, which offers universal coverage, as an example of a program with basic provisions (Evans, 1989). The proposal modeled on Canada's is for entitlement of a range of comprehensive services from a doctor's visit, prescription drugs, and even nursing home care. The Canadian system does have some imposed limitations and waiting lists for elective care, but it provides basic and emergency care to everyone at about 7% of G.N.P. in contrast to 12% of the United States G.N.P. Health care experts tell us that Canadian health care is comparable to our own. The first objective of any national health policy is the elimination of financial barriers to health care services.

There is talk of the need to ration health care given our limited financial resources. It is clear that we cannot provide everything to everyone. There is no health care system in the world that does provide everything. In a sense we are rationing care today – geographically and economically. Certainly the 37 million uninsured or underinsured Americans have their health care rationed. There may be a need to place limitations on given medical services. However, 89% of Americans say they are concerned "by the way who gets what" in health care. They want a change (Harris Poll, 1989). They would prefer a universal coverage program rather than a multi-type private health insurance system which rations by payment. Basic and essential care – diagnostic, therapeutic, and rehabilitative – is what would be considered fair and should be equitably available. Most Americans agree that spending billions of dollars for heart transplants for a few serves as a frank denial of care to those needy children and mothers, and to those lacking access. Making decisions about what should be basic and guaranteed is not difficult. The hard fight will be to deny the special groups their special interests.

We are not suggesting that scientific investigation should be curtailed. When new technology comes to the fore, it must be assessed for its cost-effectiveness and general benefits. The introduction of the lithotripsy program which deals with the elimination of kidney stones has saved us from doing 8,000 surgical kidney procedures each year (Lamm, 1989, p. 9), even if there is some indication of the tendency for a recurrence of stones. In contrast, medicine offers renal dialysis at an overwhelming cost for known dying patients without a chance of survival, to give them a few extra days or weeks of questionable lifestyle. The choices in the use of technology and specialized treatment cannot be based on the fact that they are available, but rather that they are of demonstrated high benefit in terms of affecting functional capacities, are cost effective and can save and improve the life of many. Patients or their named surrogates should be given final choice when special determination is needed.

America needs a national health plan — a strategy that covers essential, universal coverage without financial barriers to access, is equitably and soundly financed and offers fair payment to providers, and which "encourages appropriate treatment and appropriate utilization by consumers" (The Nation's Health, July 1989, p. 8).

The President of the American Hospital Association says "any supportable reform proposal should be able to sustain a rational continuum of health care services that are:

— Of high quality;
— Community focused;
— In sufficient supply of timely access;
— Efficiently delivered;
— Conducive to innovation;
— Adequately and fairly financed;
— Affordable; and
— As far as essential services are concerned, available to all"
  (Hospitals, August 20, 1989, pp. 26-27).

We agree with the standards suggested by McCarthy but inject some other vital considerations.

The national health plan will need to include professional accountability measures while it assures effective and efficient organization of services and their quality. Government at all levels will need to have major roles to safeguard the public and to assure health care providers' responsiveness to the people's needs. A basic tenet of a national health plan is the recognition that medical care is not health care. Social-health services include the prevention of diseases of all types and health promotion, even though the benefits from prevention still need to be demonstrated (Russell, 1985). Stevens suggests that the study of health education and health maintenance programs needs to include the variables of the quality of life and the social costs to patients and families when assessing cost-effectiveness (Stevens, 1985). The assessment of quality of life (q.o.l.) and patient satisfaction as a result of care are now seen as two measurements to judge the outcome of service (Patrick and Erickson, 1988).

Prevention and health maintenance programs are generally multi-professional in design, and are best administered by the most appropriately equipped professional, using consultation and team interaction when needed. We have noted that social-health care cannot continue to be medicalized care. The more doctors we have, the more doctor visits we will have. Lamm noted that every 'excess' doctor in practice increases the Nation's health costs by $300,000 annually or $12 million over 40 years (Lamm, 1989, p. 5) because a doctor will support medical visits to his office, in the same way that hospitals need to keep their beds filled. Visits and occupied beds are income producing, but not necessarily the most valid mode of care.

People tend to use doctors to deal with any ailment they may have, whether socially, psychologically, or environmentally induced. While symptoms may well be physical or emotional in nature, "the burden of treatment is placed on the least equipped of the providers" (Rehr and Miller, 1983, p. 258). More doctors, more hospital beds, more technology will not change the social ailments of the populations-at-risk. It is more evident to most health care professionals, to many doctors, as well as to the lay public that a biomedical focus does not help to alleviate the problems of stress, anxiety, depression, worry, and a host of social ailments, social diseases, and environmentally-induced symptoms. What is needed, is policy and planning that allows the assignment of essential services to appropriate providers, such as social problems to social workers, prevention to nurses and/or to health educators, and mental health counseling to trained counselors rather than to the most expensive and least equipped physicians.

We need to rethink the commercialization of hospitals. Hospitals are social and public utilities, and to privatize them without holding the for-profit institution responsible for care to all as the nonprofit is, is a denial of service. As we recognize the changing patterns in health care delivery, the roles and functions of health care professionals and personnel will change as well. We shall need to be responsive to changes in the training and education of health care workers while we examine the power of guilds to protect their turf.

Today there is more and more feeling of loss of control within the practice of a professional within his own profession, and certainly in diminishing collaboration. Bureaucratization, paperwork, regulation oversight, and monitoring contribute to the growing dissatisfaction in assuming a personal health care profession. There is open acknowledgement that today's health professionals have not been educated to deal with the changing care needs.

A sound social welfare program will need to be incorporated into the national health plan with recognition that they go together, and that a range of skills provided by different professionals will be required to contribute to social-health maintenance. A national health plan is one that is social-health in character and as such is multi-disciplinary, collaborative and cooperative, and supportive of each profession's contributions to patient care. It requires the development of skilled workers, a redefinition of jobs so that there is status and financial reward for all health care workers, as well as upward mobility tracks (Morris, 1989).

Educating the consumers of health care would be a major component of a national health plan. In addition to learning their rights and their responsibilities, consumers will have to become knowledgeable about health care and what it takes to deliver sound, efficient, and effective services. When consumers are knowledgeable about health care, they will be able to join with providers, and with key parties in the public and private sectors to create a partnership in evaluating care, in planning to improve the delivery of services, and in grappling with ethical problems. While ethical dilemmas will be struggled out in the context of the social good, the individual good can also be recognized. The individual consumer will also need to learn to play an active role in his own health status. When ill, a partnership between doctor and consumer can make for more intelligent decision-making, since each can assume a role supportive of motivation for essential self care.

It may seem strange that two health care professionals should now make a plea for change in our public educational system, a system which currently may be the second biggest deterrent to safeguarding the social welfare, and the quality of life and health care in the United States. We have a failing educational system, unable to teach its students to become productive and knowledgeable members of society. The quality of teachers, the limited supply, havoc in the classroom, chaos in inner city classrooms have led to low proficiency, illiteracy, and a group of youngsters finishing school unable or unwilling to participate in the labor force, and unable to care for themselves in support of the quality of their own life. Self-destructive behavior in our youth is beyond the scope of the medical establishment. It needs to be addressed in social, familial, and educational terms. Yet, without an educated youth, no health gains can be safeguarded in the future. Our best minds must deal with the challenge of educating today's and tomorrow's children.

Research, both scientific and applied, is a critical component of national health planning. Research today is frequently too politically oriented. We need researched data for planning. Scientific achievements will continue with the support of government and private industry. Most important to the deliberations of national health policy and planning is making available adequate, sound information governing populations-at-risk, the health care delivery, cost-effective programs and treatments, and professional performance and service outcomes, along with data on the range of social and health problems we have noted. Such data need to be available at regional planning levels, where coalitions of business, government, insurers, providers, academics, and consumers can deal with them for resource deliberations for local needs. Applied studies for the enhancement of practice is what the clinicians seek from the researchers.

Will we have a national social-health policy and an operational plan? The public wants it; industry wants it; the unions want it. We must convince our government representatives that universal access to a comprehensive and quality based health care system is both the desire, and in the interest of all Americans. A rational social-health policy and plan will take intensive, on-going and hard choice deliberations among a group of statesmanlike providers, consumers and politicians who are knowledgeable, who have available to them sound and current information and data, and who believe in an equitable and just system of care for all Americans.

REFERENCES

AHA, *Washington Watch*, April/May 1990.

V.A. Ancona-Berk and T.C. Chalmers, "An Analysis of the Costs of Ambulatory and Inpatient Care," *American Journal of Public Health*, 76(9), September 1986, pp. 1102-1104.

Joseph A. Califano, Jr., "Millions Blown in Health," *New York Times*, April 12, 1989.

Karen Davis, "Access to Health Care in a Cost-Conscious Society," *Access to Social-Health Care*, ed. by H. Rehr, Ginn Press, 1986, pp. 23-53.

Carrol L. Estes, "Aging, Health, and Social Policy: Crisis and Crossroads," *Journal of Aging and Social Policy*, Vol. 1(1/2), 1989, pp. 17-31.

Robert G. Evans et al., "Controlling Health Expenditures: The Canadian Reality," *New England Journal of Medicine*, 320(9), 1989, pp. 571-577.

Melvin A. Glasser, "Access to Social-Health Care: Who Shall Decide What? Impact on Consumers," *Access to Social-Health Care*, ed. by H. Rehr, Ginn Press, 1986, pp. 63-70.

Harris Poll, 1989.

Hospitals, May 5, 1988, July 5, 1989, pp. 52-54, and August 20, 1989, pp. 14 and 25.

Marc Lalonde, *A New Perspective on the Health of Canadians*, Information Canada, 1975, pp. 38-50.

Richard D. Lamm, "Columbus and Copernicus: New Wine in Old Wineskins," *Mount Sinai Journal of Medicine*, 56(1), Jan. 1989, pp. 1-10.

Philip Longman, "Social Security and the Baby Boom Generation," *Journal of Aging and Social Policy*, 1(1/2), 1989, pp. 131-153.

Marc M. Melum, "Hospitals Must Change, Control is the Issue," *Hospitals*, March 1, 1989, pp. 67-72.

A.R. Meyers and R.J. Masters, "Managed Care for High Risk Populations," *Journal of Aging and Social Policy*, 1(1/2), 1989.

Rosalind S. Miller, "Legislation and Health Policies," *Social Work Issues in Health Care,* ed. by R.S. Miller and H. Rehr, Prentice-Hall, N.J., 1983, pp. 74-120.

Robert Morris, "Challenges of Aging in Tomorrow's World: Will Gerontology Grow, Stagnate or Change?" *The Gerontologist*, 29(4), 1989, pp. 494-501.

National Center for Health Statistics, unpublished data, 1988.

D.L. Patrick and P. Erickson, "What constitutes quality of life? Concepts and dimensions," *Quality of Life and Cardiovascular Care*, 1988, 4:103-127.

Helen Rehr, "More Issues in the Eighties," *Social Work Issues in Health Care,* ed. by R.S. Miller and H. Rehr, Prentice-Hall, N.J., 1983, pp. 252-277.

Helen Rehr and Gary Rosenberg, "Access to Social-Health Care: Implications for Social Work," *Access to Social-Health Care*, ed. by H. Rehr, Ginn Press, 1986, pp. 77-78.

Arnold S. Relman, "The New Medical-Industrial Complex," *New England Journal of Medicine*, 1980, 303:963-970.

James B. Reuler, "Health Care for the Homeless in a National Health Program," *American Journal of Public Health*, Aug. 1989, 79(8), pp. 1033-1035.

William Ruddick, "Why Not a General Right to Health Care," *Mount Sinai Journal of Medicine*, 56(3), May 1989.

Lois Russell, "Cost-Effectiveness and Prevention," presentation at Community Medicine Grand Rounds, Mount Sinai School of Medicine, NY, Jan. 18, 1985.

Rosemary Stevens, "The Changing Hospital," presentation at Community Medicine Grand Rounds, Mount Sinai School of Medicine, NY, Feb. 15, 1985.

The Nation's Health, "APHA Board Endorses Criteria for a National Health Plan," July 1989, p. 8.

Lewis Thomas, "On the Science and Technology of Medicine," *Daedalus*, Winter 1977.

J.M. Weiner, R.J. Hanley, D.A. Spence and S.E. Murray, "We Can Run But We Can't Hide: Toward Reforming Long-Term Care," *Journal of Aging and Social Policy*, 1(1/2), 1989, pp. 87-102.

APPENDIXES

APPENDIX A:
THE DORIS SIEGEL MEMORIAL FUND COMMITTEE

Honorary Chairmen
   Dr. Thomas C. Chalmers
   Dr. S. David Pomrinse
   Dr. John W. Rowe

Committee

   Mrs. Susan S. Bailis
   Mrs. Robert M. Benjamin
   Dr. Barbara Berkman
   Mr. Philip Bernstein
   Dr. Susan Blumenfield
   Dr. Lawrence Cuzzi
   Mrs. Bess Dana
   Dr. Kurt W. Deuschle
   Dr. Sally Faith Dorfman
   Ms. Kathy Forrest
   Dr. Valentin Fuster
   Dr. Alex Gitterman
   Dr. Richard Gorlin
   Dr. Katherine Grimm
   Mrs. Gail G. Grob
   Mrs. Celia Hailperin
   Dr. Joseph M. Hassett

   Mrs. Walter A. Hirsch*
   Dr. Karen Kaplan
   Mrs. Seymour M. Klein*
   Mrs. Robert A. Levinson
   Mrs. Jane Isaacs Lowe
   Michael G. Macdonald, Esq.
   Mrs. Jane B. Mayer
   Miss Janice Paneth
   Mrs. Marjorie Pleshette
   Dr. Helen Rehr
   Dr. David Rose
   Dr. Maurice V. Russell
   Mrs. Beatrice P. Sachs
   Mrs. Marvin H. Schur
   Dr. Cecil Sheps
   Dr. Harry Spiera
   Mrs. Elinor Stevens
   Miss Judith Trachtenberg
   Mrs. Frank L. Weil
   Dr. Gail Kuhn Weissman
   Mrs. Mary Wolf
   Dr. Alma T. Young

Executive Secretary
   Dr. Gary Rosenberg

---

*deceased

APPENDIX B:
SUB-COMMITTEE ON PLANNING

Dr. Samuel J. Bosch
Mrs. Bess Dana
Mrs. Gail G. Grob
Mrs. Robert A. Levinson
Miss Janice Paneth
Mrs. Marjorie Pleshette
Dr. Helen Rehr
Dr. Gary Rosenberg

Dr. Maurice V. Russell
Mrs. Beatrice P. Sachs
Mrs. Marvin H. Schur
Dr. Alma T. Young

Staff

Ms. Susan Crimmins

APPENDIX C: WORKSHOPS

I. Delivery of Clinical Personal Health Services

Leader: Professor Rosalind Miller
Recorder: Mrs. Zelda Foster
Presenters:
1. Dr. Carol H. Meyer, "The Changing Demography and Nature of Health Care Problems";
2. Ms. Diana Katz, "Engaging the Consumer";
3. Dr. Mack Lipkin, Jr., "Collaborative Relationships."

II. Organization and Management of Social-Health Resources

Co-Leaders: Dr. Andrew Weissman and Mr. Ray Cornbill
Recorder: Dr. Lawrence Cuzzi
Presenters:
1. Ms. Ruth Breslin, "Reconciling Past, Present, and Future";
2. Dr. Katherine Grimm, "Collaborative Relationships Among Health Care Professions";
3. Dr. David Saunders, "Reconciling Cost-Effectiveness with Optimum Social-Health Outcomes";
4. Ms. Linda McGoldrick, "Impact of Auspices, Reimbursement, and Financing Patterns on Health Care Problems."

III. Health Policy, Planning, and Regulations

Leader: Ms. Myrna Lewis
Recorder: Ms. Barbara Brenner
Presenters:
1. Mr. Herbert Lukashok, "Reconciling Cost-Effectiveness with Optimum Social-Health Outcomes";
2. Dr. Michael Mulvihill, "Changing Demography and Nature of Health Problems";
3. Dr. Charlotte Muller, "Impact of Auspices, Reimbursement, and Financing Patterns on Health Care Problems."

IV. Education of Health Care Professions

Co-Leaders: Dr. Phyllis Caroff and Dr. Joseph Hassett
Recorder: Ms. Jane I. Lowe
Presenters:
1. Dr. Thomas Carlton, "Reconciling Past, Present, and Future";
2. Dr. David Cohen, "Impact of Social-Health Policy Changes on Education for the Health Professions";
3. Dr. Howard Zucker, "Preparing the Health Care Professions for Changing Health Needs."

V. Research and Evaluation

Leader: Dr. Gerard Reardon
Recorder: Dr. Nancy Showers
Presenters:
1. Dr. Barbara Berkman, "Reconciling Past, Present, and Future";
2. Dr. James McTigue, "Changing Demography and the Nature of Health Care Problems";
3. Dr. Hans Falck, "Multi-Disciplinary Approaches to Research";
4. Dr. Marianne C. Fahs, "Reconciling Cost-Effectiveness with Optimum Social-Health Outcomes."

APPENDIX D: PARTICIPANTS

Marcia Abramson, DSW
Assistant Professor
Columbia University School of Social Work
New York, NY

Patricia Anvaripour, RN, CNAA
Planning Associate
Department of Nursing
Mount Sinai Medical Center
New York, NY

Gerald N. Beallor, MSW
Director
Department of Social Work Services
Montefiore Medical Center
Bronx, NY

Candyce Berger, PhD
Director
Department of Social Work Services
University Hospital
Seattle, WA

Barbara Berkman, DSW
Professor and Director of Research and Quality Assurance
Department of Social Work Services
Massachusetts General Hospital
Boston, MA

Susan Blumenfield, DSW
Assistant Professor and Director
Department of Social Work Services
Mount Sinai Medical Center
New York, NY

Evelyn Bonander, MSW
  Director
  Department of Social Work Services
  Massachusetts General Hospital
  Boston, MA

Barbara Brenner, MSW
  Director
  Department of Community Relations
  Mount Sinai Medical Center
  New York, NY

Ruth Breslin, MSW
  Chief Social Worker
  Yale-New Haven Hosptial
  New Haven, CT

Eleanor Brilliant, DSW
  Associate Professor and Director
  Undergraduate Social Work Program
  Rutgers University School of Social Work
  New Brunswick, NJ

Diana Brown, CSW
  Director
  Department of Social Work Services
  Tisch Hospital
  New York, NY

Thomas Carlton, DSW
  Professor
  School of Social Work
  Virginia Commonwealth University
  Richmond, VA

Phyllis Caroff, DSW
  Professor
  School of Social Work
  Hunter College
  New York, NY

Esther Chachkes, MSW
    Director
    Department of Social Work Services
    Presbyterian Hospital
    New York, NY

Sylvia Clarke, MSW
    Consultant
    Department of Social Work Services
    The Mount Sinai Medical Center, and
    Editor
    Social Work in Health Care

David Cohen, MD
    Director
    Ambulatory Care Services
    Mount Sinai Medical Center
    New York, NY

Ray Cornbill, MBA
    Executive Vice President
    North General Hospital
    New York, NY

Lawrence Cuzzi, DSW
    Director
    Department of Social Work Services
    City Hospital at Elmhurst
    Queens, NY

Bess Dana, MSW
    Professor Emerita
    Department of Community Medicine
    Mount Sinai School of Medicine
    New York, NY

Kurt W. Deuschle, MD
    Chairman and Professor
    Department of Community Medicine
    Mount Sinai School of Medicine
    New York, NY

Cynthia Dortz, MSW
Instructor
Department of Community Medicine
Mount Sinai School of Medicine
New York, NY

Golda M. Edinburg, MSW
Director
Department of Social Work Services
McLean Hospital Division
Massachusetts General Hospital
Belmont, MA

Marianne Fahs, MPH, PhD
Assistant Professor and Associate Director
Division of Health Economics
Department of Community Medicine
Mount Sinai School of Medicine
New York, NY

Hans S. Falck, PhD
Professor
School of Social Work
Virginia Commonwealth University
Richmond, VA

Howard Fillitt, MD
Associate Professor
Department of Geriatrics
Mount Sinai School of Medicine
New York, NY

Mary Foley, EdD
Instructor
Department of Community Medicine (Social Work)
Mount Sinai School of Medicine
New York, NY

Zelda Foster, MSW
  Chief
  Department of Social Work Services
  V.A. Medical Center
  Brooklyn, NY

David Freed, MBA
  Vice President
  Support Services
  The Mount Sinai Hospital
  New York, NY

Emily Friedman, BA
  Contributing Editor
  Medical World News,
  Health Care Forum Journal,
  Hospitals,
  Health Business, and
  Contributing Writer
  JAMA

George S. Getzel, DSW
  Professor
  School of Social Work
  Hunter College
  New York, NY

Katherine Teats-Grimm, MD
  Associate Professor of Clinical Pediatrics
  Department of Pediatrics
  Mount Sinai School of Medicine
  New York, NY

Trude Gruber, MSW
  Teaching Assistant
  Department of Community Medicine (Social Work)
  Mount Sinai School of Medicine
  New York, NY

Joseph Hassett, MD
Assistant Professor
Department of Medicine
Mount Sinai School of Medicine
New York, NY

Audreye Johnson, PhD
Associate Professor
School of Social Work
University of North Carolina-Chapel Hill
Chapel Hill, NC

Michael Katch, DSW
Assistant Director
Department of Social Work Services
City Hospital at Elmhurst
Queens, NY

Diana Katz, MBA
Consumer Member
Community Board
Mount Sinai Medical Center
New York, NY

A. Donna King, MSW
Director
Department of Social Work Services
Health Key Medical Group
St. Louis, MO

Stanley J. Kissell*
Chief
Department of Social Work Services
National Institute of Health
Bethesda, MD

*deceased

Lorraine Levy, MSW
Assistant Director
Department of Social Work Services
City Hospital at Elmhurst
Queens, NY

Myrna Lewis, MS
Instructor
Department of Community Medicine (Social Work)
Mount Sinai School of Medicine
New York, NY

Mack Lipkin, Jr., MD
Director, Primary Care,
Internal Medicine and Pediatric Residency
New York University School of Medicine
New York, NY

Hannah Lipsky, MSW
Lecturer
Department of Community Medicine (Social Work)
Mount Sinai School of Medicine
New York, NY

Herbert Lukashok, MS
Associate Professor and Vice-Chairman
Department of Epidemiology and Social Medicine
Albert Einstein College of Medicine
Bronx, NY

Jane I. Lowe, MS
Instructor
Department of Community Medicine (Social Work)
Mount Sinai School of Medicine
New York, NY

Linda McGoldrick, MSW, MBA
Managing Director
Financial Health Associates
New York, NY

James F. McTigue, PhD
  Associate Director
  National Center of Social Policy and Practice
  Silver Spring, MD

Jane B. Mayer, MSW
  Director
  Department of Social Work Services
  Beth Israel Hospital
  Boston, MA

Carol H. Meyer, DSW
  Professor
  School of Social Work
  Columbia University
  New York, NY

Rosalind Miller, MSW
  Associate Professor
  School of Social Work
  Columbia University
  New York, NY

Terry Mizrahi, PhD
  Professor
  School of Social Work
  Hunter College
  New York, NY

Charlotte Muller, PhD
  Director
  Division of Health Economics
  Department of Community Medicine
  Mount Sinai School of Medicine
  New York, NY

Michael Mulvihill, DrPH
  Associate Professor
  Department of Geriatrics and Adult Development
  Mount Sinai School of Medicine
  New York, NY

Elizabeth Murphy, RN
Assistant Director
Department of Nursing
Mount Sinai Medical Center
New York, NY

Dennis O'Leary, MD
President
Joint Commission on Accreditation
of Health Organizations
Chicago, IL

Gerard Reardon, DSW
Assistant Professor
Department of Community Medicine (Social Work)
Mount Sinai School of Medicine
New York, NY

Helen Rehr, DSW
Professor Emerita
Department of Community Medicine (Social Work)
Mount Sinai School of Medicine
New York, NY

Barry Rock, DSW
Director
Department of Social Work Services
Long Island Jewish Medical Center
New Hyde Park, NY

Gary Rosenberg, PhD
Edith J. Baerwald Professor
Department of Community Medicine (Social Work)
Mount Sinai School of Medicine
New York, NY

Beatrice Phillips Sachs, MS
Member
Doris Siegel Memorial Fund Committee

David Saunders, PhD
  Professor
  School of Social Work
  Virginia Commonwealth University
  Richmond, VA

Joel Seligman, MBA
  Assistant Director
  Mount Sinai Medical Center
  New York, NY

Vivian Shapiro, MSW
  Research Associate
  Department of Community Medicine (Social Work)
  Mount Sinai School of Medicine
  New York, NY

Nancy Showers, DSW
  Teaching Assistant
  Department of Community Medicine (Social Work)
  Mount Sinai School of Medicine
  New York, NY

Mary Ellen Siegel, MSW
  Teaching Assistant
  Department of Community Medicine (Social Work)
  Mount Sinai School of Medicine
  New York, NY

Ellen Simon, DSW
  Director
  Department of Social Work Service
  Beth Abraham Hospital
  Bronx, NY

Zvi Stern, MD
  Associate Director
  Hadassah Medical Center
  Jerusalem, Israel

Leonard Tuzman, CSW
Associate Director
Department of Social Work Services
Long Island Jewish Medical Center
New Hyde Park, NY

Virginia Walther, MSW
Teaching Assistant
Department of Comunity Medicine (Social Work)
Mount Sinai School of Medicine
New York, NY

Lois Weinstein, MA
Director
Program Planning
Memorial Hospital
New York, NY

Andrew Weissman, PhD
Director
ALTRO Health and Rehabilitation Services
New York, NY

Richard Woodrow, DSW
Associate Director, Field Work,
and Assistant Professor
School of Social Work
Columbia University
New York, NY

Alma T. Young, EdD
Assistant Professor
Department of Community Medicine (Social Work)
Mount Sinai School of Medicine
New York, NY

Ilise Zimmerman, MPH, MBA
Assistant Director
Mount Sinai Medical Center
New York, NY

Howard Zucker, MD
Lecturer
Department of Medicine
Mount Sinai School of Medicine
New York, NY

Index